MRCS Revision Guide: Limbs and Spine

MRCS Revision Guide: Limbs and Spine

Mazyar Kanani, PhD, FRCS (CTh)
Fellow in Congenital Cardiac Surgery, Children's Hospital, Pittsburgh, Pennsylvania, USA

Khaled M. Sarraf, BSc (Hons), MBBS, MRCS
Specialist Registrar in Trauma and Orthopaedic Surgery,
North West Thames Rotation – London Deanery,
Chelsea and Westminster Hospital NHS Foundation Trust, London, UK

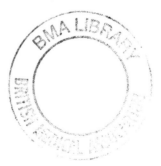

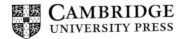
CAMBRIDGE
UNIVERSITY PRESS

CAMBRIDGE UNIVERSITY PRESS
Cambridge, New York, Melbourne, Madrid, Cape Town,
Singapore, São Paulo, Delhi, Mexico City

Cambridge University Press
The Edinburgh Building, Cambridge CB2 8RU, UK

Published in the United States of America
by Cambridge University Press, New York

www.cambridge.org
Information on this title: www.cambridge.org/9780521139762

First published 2012

Printed in the United Kingdom at the University Press, Cambridge

A catalogue record for this publication is available from the British Library

Library of Congress Cataloguing-in-Publication Data

Kanani, Mazyar.
  MRCS revision guide: limbs and spine / Mazyar Kanani, Khaled M. Sarraf.
    p.   cm.
  ISBN 978-0-521-13976-2 (Paperback)
  1. Spine–Surgery–Examinations, questions, etc.   2. Extremities (Anatomy)–
Surgery–Examinations, questions, etc.   3. Royal College of Surgeons of England.
  I. Sarraf, Khaled M.   II. Title.
  RD768.K36 2012
  617.4'710076–dc23   2011039825

ISBN 978-0-521-13976-2 Paperback

To my parents and brother for their endless support and my wife, Bana, for her patience in enduring the long hours put into writing this book.
KMS

For Carl Kanani.
MK

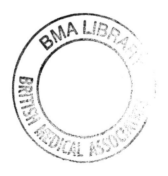

Contents

Section 2 Examinations

Preface

"President Kennedy said that an error becomes a mistake only when you refuse to correct it."

Vigilance is the only tool we have to manage the errors that lurk around each hospital corridor. It is hoped that this book will not only help prepare for the challenges of the new MRCS exam, but also help keep our clinical vigilance honed and ready for the supreme challenge – our sick patients.

Mazyar Kanani and Khaled M. Sarraf

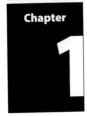

Applied surgical science

Action potentials

What is meant by the 'equilibrium potential' for an ion?

The equilibrium potential for an ion is the potential difference at which that ion ceases to flow across the cell membrane. It is calculated using the *Nernst* equation.

What is meant by the 'resting membrane potential' for a cell?

This is the potential difference across the cell membrane. It forms because of the ionic fluxes of Na^+, K^+ and Cl^- across the membrane, the sizes of which are determined by their electrochemical gradients.

What is the typical value of the resting membrane potential for neuron?

A typical value is -70 mV. The value is negative because the interior of the cell is negatively charged with respect to the exterior.

What is the importance of the Na^+/K^+ pump for the equilibrium potential?

This pump, which is ATPase-driven, transports three Na^+ ions out of the cell for every two K^+ ions pumped in. It helps to maintain the internal and external ionic environment, which progressively alters as ions naturally flow down their electrochemical gradients. In doing so, it maintains and sustains the potential difference across the cell (the resting membrane potential).

What is an action potential? Draw and label the axes of a typical action potential for a neuron

An action potential (Figure 1.1) is defined as the rapid change in the membrane potential (depolarization) that occurs following stimulation of an excitable cell. It is followed by a rapid return to the resting membrane potential (repolarization).

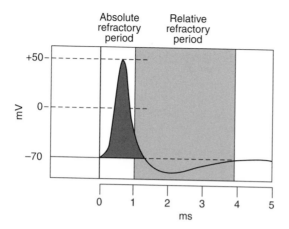

Figure 1.1 An action potential.

- Note that depolarization is an 'all-or-none' response, in that the action potential is generated only when the threshold potential is produced by the stimulus. Subthreshold stimuli do not generate the action potential.

- For any individual excitable cell, each action potential is of the same amplitude, and propagated at the same speed.

Briefly describe the ionic basis for the action potential

The changes in the fluxes of ions that account for depolarization are shown in Figure 1.2.

- Once the threshold potential is reached by the stimulus, the voltage-sensitive Na^+ channels open, causing a rapid influx of Na^+ ions into the cell. This causes depolarization, and the membrane potential becomes positive. Once open, the Na^+ channel closes again within a millisecond.

- During the initial opening of the Na^+ channels, a positive feedback loop is initiated; so more channels open up, leading to rapid depolarization.

- The cell would remain depolarized if it were not for the rapid closure (inactivation) of the Na^+ channels.

- At the same time, there is a constant background movement of K^+ ions out of the cell. This has the effect of placing a limit on the change of membrane potential during the depolarization phase of the action potential.

- During repolarization, there is the opening of the voltage-sensitive K^+ channels, leading to loss of K^+ from the cell. These react more slowly

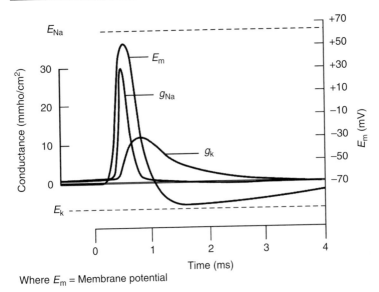

Where E_m = Membrane potential

Figure 1.2 Depolarization and repolarization in an action potential.

than the Na^+ channels, and are open for longer. Thus, repolarization, with a return to the resting membrane potential is a slower process than depolarization.

- After lots of action potentials, when there is the exchange of many ions, the ionic environment is returned to the steady state by the continued and persistent action of the Na^+/K^+ pumps.

What is meant by 'refractory period'?

This is the temporary state immediately after an action potential when no further action potential may be initiated. It can be divided into two parts:

Absolute refractory period	The first stage of this phase, when no action potential may be generated, irrespective of the amplitude of the stimulus.
Relative refractory period	The latter part of this phase, when the cell membrane may be brought to threshold only with a larger-than-normal stimulus.

What is the effect of myelination on a nerve fibre?

Myelination fibres have their axons enveloped with the myelin and cell bodies of a Schwann's cell (or oligodendrocyte in the CNS). This has a number of effects on the propagation of action potentials along the axons of the myelinated neurons, compared with unmyelinated ones:

The conduction velocity is increased	The large fibres of the myelinated neuron have lower resistance to current flow, owing to a larger number of intracellular ions.
Saltatory conditions	Current is generated only at the nodes of Ranvier, and not at the myelin sheath. Consequently, the current *jumps* quickly between nodes, reducing the time for delivery of signals.

What types of nerve fibre are there?

Peripheral nerve fibres may be classified in the following way:

Group A -- These are the largest (up to 20 µm).

α (Ia and Ib)	motor and proprioception fibres,
β (II)	Touch, pressure and proprioception fibres,
γ (II)	Muscle spindle fusimotor fibres,
δ (III)	Touch, pain and pressure fibres.

Group B -- Myelinated fibres, which are autonomic preganglionic (up to 3 µm).

Group C (Type IV) -- Unmyelinated fibres, which carry postganglionic fibres, and fibres for touch and pain (up to 2 µm).

How do local anaesthetic agents alter the conduction along a neuron?

Some agents can modify the activation and propagation of the action potential. Local anaesthetic agents are composed of an amine group connected to an aromatic side chain via an ester or amide bond. They are selective blockers of the voltage-dependant Na^+ channels.

Arterial pressure

Draw the arterial pressure waveform, and label the axes

The arterial pressure waveform is shown in Figure 1.3. The 'dicrotic notch' is a momentary rise in the arterial pressure trace following closure of the aortic valve.

How is the mean arterial pressure (MAP) calculated from this waveform?

The mean arterial pressure (MAP) is calculated by dividing the area under the pressure wave by the time measured.

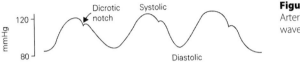

Figure 1.3
Arterial pressure waveform.

How may the MAP be calculated simply?

$$MAP = \text{Diastolic pressure} + 1/3(\text{Systolic pressure} - \text{Diastolic pressure}).$$

Why is the mean pressure not a simple average of the systolic and diastolic pressures?

This is because the mean pressure is time-weighted; for about two-thirds of the time cycle, the pressure is close to the diastolic level.

What is blood pressure (BP)?

This is defined as the product of the cardiac output (CO) and the systemic vascular resistance (SVR),

$$BP = CO \times SVR,$$

where the cardiac output is the product of the heart rate (HR) and the stroke volume (SV):

$$CO = HR \times SV.$$

How does the arterial pressure waveform at the aortic root differ from that further distally in the arterial tree? Why is this?

Figure 1.4 shows pressure waveforms at the aortic root and further along the arterial tree. These differences are in part due to the changes in wall stiffness along the arterial tree, and their consequent effects on the transmission of the pulse wave along the vessel.

What are the two basic mechanisms involved in the control of the arterial pressure?

Short-term regulation by neuronal pathways involving a multineuronal reflex arc consisting of receptors, afferent pathways and effectors.

Long-term regulation by the control of the extracellular fluid (ECF) volume. This is especially important after a period of fluid depletion.

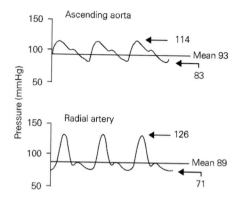

Figure 1.4 Pressure waves at different sites in the arterial tree. With transmission of the pressure wave into the distal aorta and large arteries, the systolic pressure increases and the diastolic pressure decreases, with a resultant heightening of the pulse pressure waveform. However, the mean pressure declines steadily.

Calcium haemostasis and vitamin D metabolism

What is the normal serum calcium concentration?

The calcium level should always be corrected for albumin concentration, as it is bound to it, and its range is 2.2–2.6 mmol/l.

What is the approximate distribution of calcium in the body?

- 99% is found in bone (mostly as hydroxyapatite),
- 0.9% is intracellular,
- 0.1% is extracellular.

In what state is calcium found in the circulation?

- 50% is unbound and ionized,
- 45% is bound to plasma proteins,
- 5% is associated with anions, such as citrate and lactate.

How is serum calcium concentration affected by the pH?

- Increased pH (alkalosis) leads to increased level of protein binding = decrease in serum calcium concentration,
- Decreased pH (acidosis) leads to decreased level of protein binding = increase in serum calcium concentration,

This explains why in hyperventilation (where there is a decrease in PCO_2 thus an increase in pH) there is an increased level of calcium bound to protein, lowering the concentration of free ionized calcium, and leading to tetany.

What is the role of calcium in the body?

- It is an important second messenger in several cell signalling pathways,
- It plays a key role in muscle contraction, nerve function and contributes to the coagulation cascade.

Which organs are involved in controlling serum calcium levels?

- Skeletal system,
- Kidneys,
- Gut.

Which hormones are involved in controlling serum calcium levels?

Parathyroid hormone (PTH)	Produced by parathyroid glands,
Vitamin D_3 (cholecalciferol)	Derived from the diet, ultraviolet light-mediated conversion in the skin, and hydroxylation in the liver and kidneys,
Calcitonin	Produced by the thyroid's parafollicular (C) cells.

Briefly describe the action of each

Parathyroid hormone (PTH).

In bone	Increases synthesis of enzymes that breakdown the matrix to release calcium and phosphate into the circulation. Also increases osteocytic and osteoclastic activity, leading to bone resorption.
In kidney	Increases renal phosphate secretion and decreases calcium excretion. Also increases 1-α hydroxylase activity, indirectly increasing calcium absorption.

Vitamin D_3 (cholecalciferol) -- The active metabolite $1,25(OH)_2D_3$ is formed by renal hydroxylation of $25(OH)D_3$.

In bone	Increases serum calcium while increases calcification of bone matrix. It increases osteoblastic activity and protein synthesis.
In kidney	Increases calcium and phosphate reabsorption.
In gut	Increases calcium and phosphate reabsorption.

Calcitonin -- Acts to reduce serum calcium if levels rise above 2.5 mmol/l.

In bone	Inhibits bone resorption through inhibiting osteoclastic activity
In kidney	Increases excretion of calcium, phosphate, sodium and chloride

What are the possible causes of vitamin D deficiency?

- Renal failure,
- Liver disease,
- Inadequate sunlight exposure in people with poor dietary vitamin D intake.

What are the effects of vitamin D deficiency?

| In children | Bowing of the extremities and collapse of the chest wall, resulting in rickets, |
| In adults | May give rise to bone pain, vertebral pathological fractures and stress fractures, resulting in osteomalacia. |

What are the clinical consequences of hypercalcaemia?

Bones, stones, abdominal groans and psychiatric moans.

- Bone lesions: notably bone cysts, osteitis fibrosa cystica and Brown's tumours of the bone,
- Muscle weakness,
- Renal calculi, secondary to hypercalciuria,
- Nephrocalcinosis: multifocal calcium deposits in renal parenchyma,
- Renal tubular dysfunction, leading to polyuria, polydipsia causing dehydration and, finally, renal failure,
- Abdominal pains: vomiting, constipation, risk of acute pancreatitis, dyspepsia and peptic ulceration, secondary to acid secretion stimulated by calcium and PTH,
- Fatigue, lethargy and organic psychosis.

What is the emergency management of hypercalcaemia?

Acute hypercalcaemia (3.0–3.5 mmol/l) involves:

- Treating underlying cause,
- Commencing cardiac monitoring,
- Rehydration with crystalloid – Frusemide can be added to help in calcium dieresis,
- Bisphosphonate infusion can rapidly reduce serum calcium, e.g. pamidronate,
- Calcitonin has a shorter duration of action (rarely used),
- High dose steroid in cases such as myeloma or sarcoidosis,
- Urgent surgery if cause is hyperparathyroidism.

What are the clinical consequences of hypocalcaemia?

- Neuromuscular irritability presenting as peripheral or circumoral paraesthesia,
- Muscular cramps,
- Tetany,

- Clinical signs:
  - Chvostek's sign: Twitching of facial muscles on tapping of the facial nerve,
  - Trousseau's sign: Tetanic spasms of hand after blood-pressure-cuff-induced ischaemia.

What is the emergency management of hypocalcaemia?

- Treat underlying cause,
- Commence cardiac monitoring,
- Adequate fluid resuscitation,
- 10 ml of 10% calcium gluconate immediately, followed by 10–40 ml in a saline infusion over 4–8 h (follow hospital protocol),
- Re-check calcium levels,
- Consider commencing oral calcium and vitamin D early.

What is the most important surgical cause of hypocalcaemia?

- Inadvertent removal of the parathyroid glands in thyroid surgery,
- Treatment with calcium and vitamin D, one or two days prior to parathyroid surgery may help prevent the development of severe hypocalcaemia.

Cartilage

What is cartilage?

Cartilage is a flexible connective tissue found in various parts of the body.

What are the types of cartilage?

Elastic cartilage	found in the outer ear and larynx.
Fibrocartilage	found in tendons, pubic symphysis, annulus fibrosus of the intervertebral disc, and menisci (fibroelastic type). Fibrocartilage contains Type I and II collagen.
Hyaline cartilage	articular cartilage.

What is the composition of articular cartilage?

Approximately 1% chondrocytes and 99% matrix. Chondrocytes are responsible for protein synthesis. They produce collagen and proteoglycans and release enzymes to break down aging components.

The matrix is made up of

Water (~70%) — Allows for lubrication and nutrition of the cartilage,

Collagen, mainly Type II (~15%) — Framework that provides tensile strength,

Proteoglycans (~15%) — Provides the cartilage resiliency to compression.

How does the anatomy of the articular cartilage affect its healing?

Unlike other connective tissues, cartilage does not contain blood vessels. Therefore, healing is limited and slow. The chondrocytes are supplied by diffusion, which is aided by the action generated from compression of the articular cartilage during movement of the joint.

Superficial cartilage injury does not cross the tidemark of the cartilage where chondrocytes can proliferate, thus cartilage does not heal.

Deep cartilage injury extends beyond the tidemark. These injuries may heal with fibrocartilage (not hyaline) formed from the bone marrow's mesenchymal stem cells at the site of injury.

Cerebrospinal fluid (CSF) and cerebral blood flow

What is the volume of the CSF?

150 ml. It is produced at rate of ~500 ml per day.

Where is it produced?

Choroid plexus of the intracerebral ventricles — accounts for 70% of production,

Blood vessels lining ventricular walls — accounts for 30% of production.

Briefly describe the CSF circulation

- From the lateral ventricle, the CSF flows into the third ventricles by way of the interventricular foramen of Monro.
- From the third ventricles, it flows into the fourth through the aqueduct of Sylvius.
- Some of the CSF then passes into the central canal of the spinal cord as a continuation of the fourth ventricle.
- The majority flows from the fourth ventricle into the subarachnoid space of the spinal cord through the central foramen of Magendie and the two laterally placed foramina of Luschka.
- After going around the spinal cord, it enters the cranial cavity through the foramen magnum, and flows around the subarachnoid space of the brain.

Where is the CSF finally absorbed?

The arachnoid villi   Accounts for 80% of absorption,

Spinal nerve roots   Accounts for 20% of absorption.

What are the arachnoid villi composed of?

These are formed from the fusion of arachnoid membrane and the endothelium of a dural venous sinus, into which it bulges.

What is the rate of cerebral blood flow?

50 ml per 100 g of brain tissue. It accounts for 15% of the cardiac output, or about 750 ml/min.

How does this rate of flow vary with arterial pressure?

The rate of flow remains essentially stable, owing to local autoregulation of flow. This is a characteristic feature of some specialized vascular beds, such as the renal system.

What is the basic mechanism of autoregulation?

There are two principle mechanisms:

Myogenic response -- An increase in the arteriolar wall tension brought on by an increase in the arterial pressure stimulates contraction of mural smooth muscle cells. The resulting vasoconstriction stabilizes the flow in the face of these pressure changes.

Vasodilator 'wash-out' -- If flow is suddenly and momentarily increased by a sudden rise in the driving pressure, locally produced vasodilation mediators are washed out of the vessel, leading to vasoconstriction and a return of the flow to the steady state.

What are the main factors that govern the cerebral blood flow?

$PaCO_2$ Hypercarbia increases the cerebral flow through an increase of the $[H^+]$. The reverse occurs with hypocarbia.

PaO_2   Hypoxia produces cerebral vasodilatation, increasing the flow. This influence is less important than the effect of $PaCO_2$.

Sympathetic stimulation   Causes some vasoconstriction, but this is the least important influence.

What is meant by cerebral perfusion pressure?

This is defined as the difference between the mean arterial pressure and the intracranial pressure. It must remain above around 70 mmHg for adequate cerebral perfusion.

Given that cerebral perfusion pressure (CPP) is equal to the difference between mean arterial pressure and intracranial pressure, the danger of hypotension is that it can lead to decreased cerebral perfusion pressure (CPP).

Microcirculation

What is this equation, and what does it describe?

$$J_v = L_pS[(P_c - P_i) - \sigma(\pi_p - \pi_i)].$$

This is the *Starling equation* and it describes the factors that determine the flow of fluid (J_v) across a capillary wall's endothelium.

Movement of water into the interstitium is produced by the hydrostatic pressure gradient ($P_c - P_i$) and counteracted by the colloid osmotic gradient ($\pi_p - \pi_i$).

P_c Capillary hydrostatic pressure.

P_i Interstitial hydrostatic pressure.

π_p Colloid oncotic (osmotic) pressure (25 mmHg).

π_i Interstitial oncotic pressure.

L_p Hydraulic conductance. This is the filtration rate per unit change of pressure across the membrane.

S Surface area of vessel wall.

σ Reflection coefficient: A measure of how leaky the membrane is. The value is around 0.8, which means that only 80% of the potential oncotic pressure is exerted across the vessel wall.

What does it mean?

It states that the net filtration of water across a capillary wall is proportional to the difference between the hydraulic and osmotic forces across the vessel wall.

What are the factors that determine the capillary hydrostatic pressure (P_c) across a capillary wall?

Distance along the capillary -- There is a fall in the pressure as you go from the arterial to the venous side of the capillary, typically from 35 mmHg to 20 mmHg.

Resistance -- Of both arterioles and venules at either end of the capillary.

Gravity -- Both arterial and venous pressures increase below the heart.

How does the resistance of surrounding arterioles and venules affect the P_c of the capillary?

- The greater the resistance of the surrounding vessels, the lower the P_c.
- What is important though is the ratio of resistance of the arteriole to the venule (R_a/R_v):

- The greater the (R_a/R_v) the lower the P_c: when the arteriole is constricted, the P_c is lower and closer to the pressure in the venule.
- The lower the (R_a/R_v) the higher the P_c: when the arteriole is less constricted, its pressure has a greater influence on the P_c.
- Following from that and Starling's equation: the greater the P_c the greater the rate of filtration of water across the vessel wall into the interstitium.

What is oedema?

Abnormal accumulation of fluid in the extravascular space.

What are the two broad types?

Transudate Results from imbalances in the hydrostatic forces of the Starling equation,

Exudate Occurs following an increase in capillary permeability (therefore larger molecules).

How may they be distinguished?

The main difference is that an exudate is rich in protein and fibrinogen – which is commonly used to aid diagnosis of the aetiology.

What are the main causes?

The main causes are categorized according to the variables in the Starling equation.

Increased capillary hydrostatic pressure (P_c) –– For example, in cardiac failure, where there is peripheral dependant oedema, ascites and pulmonary oedema. Most commonly, the main culprit is an elevation in venous pressure (as in deep vein thrombosis). Increased hydrostatic pressure also arises from abnormal retention of salt and water (e.g. in renal failure).

Reduced colloid oncotic (osmotic) pressure (π_p) –– This occurs with hypoproteinaemic states, such as malnutrition, protein-losing enteropathy and nephritic syndrome.

Increased capillary permeability –– This leads to the formation of an exudate, which follows an inflammatory process where there is an immune mediated increase in the capillary permeability (also in allergic reactions).

Lymphatic occlusion –– This leads to an accumulation of fluid in the interstitial compartment, e.g. malignant occlusion following lymphatic compression or lymphadenopathy.

Apart from increased capillary permeability, how else does inflammation promote oedema?

Vasodilatation associated with inflammation increases the capillary hydrostatic pressure, which would decrease the precapillary-to-postcapillary resistance ratio (R_a/R_v).

During an inflammatory process, what are the mediators responsible for the increase in capillary permeability?

Histamine	Released from mast cells and basophils,
5-HT	From platelets,
Platelet-activating factor	From neutrophils, basophils and macrophages,
Others	$C5_a$, PGE_2 and bradykinin.

Motor control

What kind of coordinated movements does skeletal muscle contraction lead to?

- Voluntary movement,
- Reflexes,
- Maintenance of posture,
- Repetitive and rhythmical movements, e.g. breathing.

All of these types of movement are under the control of an integrated motor system.

What are the components of the motor system that initiate, coordinate and execute these movements?

The components can be thought of as forming an interactive hierarchy. They consist of:

Cerebral cortex	Consisting of the motor cortex and associated areas,
Subcortical areas	The cerebellum, basal ganglia and brainstem,
Spinal cord	Carries fibres from the cerebral cortex to motoneurons, but also has its own intrinsic reflex activity,
Motoneurons	These form the final common pathway,
Motor units	The functional contractile unit,
Receptors and afferent pathways	These sensory pathways relay information back to the other components, which can in turn adjust movement, e.g. proprioceptive movement.

Where is the motor cortex located?

At the precentral gyrus.

Where in the spinal cord are cell bodies of the motoneuron located?

In the *ventral horns* of the spinal cord. They congregate together as motor nuclei in specific parts of the ventral horn, depending on which muscle group they are supplying.

What types of motoneuron are there, and what types of skeletal muscle fibre do they innervate?

α-motoneurons	Large-diameter fibres, innervate the majority of worker fibres. They are known as *extrafusal* fibres, since they are not encased within connective tissue sheath. They have multiple dendritic processes.
γ-motoneurons	These have smaller axons than the α-motoneurons and innervate the *intrafusal* fibres of the muscle spindle.

Apart from skeletal muscle, what other connections do motoneurons make?

Motoneurons synapse with a number of other types of cell through connections on their cell bodies:

Afferent sensory fibres	For example, afferents from cutaneous receptors that mediate cutaneous reflexes.
Descending pathways	These make synaptic connections directly from higher centres. Such connections may run down in *pyramidal* or *extrapyramidal* pathways.
Interneurons	These are the most common kind of synaptic connection onto motoneurons. They may form excitatory or inhibitory connections, and so influence motoneuron activity.

Define the motor unit

This consists of a motoneuron and all of the muscle fibres that it innervates. The size of the unit varies greatly, depending on the type of muscle; large muscles that maintain posture consist of very large units with many fibres being innervated.

Note that all of the fibres in any individual unit are of the same type. Whenever a motoneuron fires, all of the muscle fibres in that unit contract.

What type of muscle fibre forms muscle spindles?

These are formed from *intrafusal* muscle fibres. Unlike regular muscle fibres, these special fibres that form spindles are located within connective tissue capsules. The ratio of regular fibres to spindle fibres varies according to the function of each muscle.

Note that such spindle fibres lie in parallel with the regular *extrafusal* fibres.

Muscle: skeletal vs. smooth

What types of muscle are there in the body?

Skeletal Striated and voluntary,

Cardiac Striated and involuntary,

Smooth Involuntary.

What is mechanical summation?

This is when the force of contraction increases through the stimulation of multiple twitch contractions whose individual forces *accumulate*. This only occurs when the muscle is stimulated to contract before it has fully relaxed from a contraction preceding it.

What happens to the fibre if there is continuous stimulation?

If the muscle is stimulated at increasing frequency, a twitch contraction becomes a long and continuous *tetanic* contraction. The force generated by tetanus is much greater than that of a twitch. The frequency required to generate a tetanic contraction is called the *tetanic frequency*.

What are the basic types of skeletal muscle fibre? Mention briefly some of their differences

Type I -- Slow twitch fibre that is also slow to fatigue. Contains a high concentration of myoglobin, e.g., soleus muscle.

Type II -- Fast twitch that also fatigue quickly. They have large reserves of glycogen as an energy source, e.g., extraocular muscle.

Draw a sarcomere and label it

See Figure 1.5.

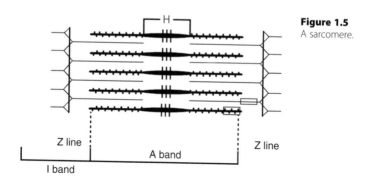

Figure 1.5
A sarcomere.

What is the function of the T tubule system, and where is it located?

This system is an invagination of the sarcolemma (muscle cell membrane). In skeletal muscle, it is located the junction of the A and I bands. It also lies adjacent to the sarcoplasmic reticulum (SR), so that there is rapid release of Ca^{2+}. It is important for the transmission of the action potential across the myofibril.

What is the source of intracellular calcium?

Calcium ions are stored in the sarcoplasmic reticulum (SR). This is a network of tubules (akin to the endoplasmic reticulum of other cells) that separates the myofibrils. The SR lies against the T tubule network. This point of contact is called the *lateral cistern* of the SR. Therefore, the action potentials running within the T tubule system can stimulate a rapid release of Ca^{2+} from the SR.

List the architectural hierarchy of the skeletal muscle cell

- The muscle is divided into bundles of fascicles that are separated by a connective tissue sheath.
- Each fascicle is composed of bundles of individual muscle fibres separated by an endomysium.
- Each muscle fibre is composed of bundles of myofibrils separated by the SR network.
- The functional unit of the myofibril is called the sarcomere. There are many of these in each myofibril, being separated at the Z line.
- The sarcomeres are formed from an arrangement of thick and thin filaments.
- The thick and thin filaments are contractile proteins.
- Thick filaments are formed from myosin.
- Thin filaments are formed from actin, troponin and tropomysin.

How does the action potential reaching the fibre finally give rise to a contraction?

The action potential brings about contraction through the process of *excitation–contraction coupling*:

- The action potential spreads out from the motor endplate through the T tubule system.
- This causes the mobilization of Ca^{2+} from the SR into the cytoplasm.
- Ca^{2+} binds to troponin C on the light chains.
- This leads to the displacement of tropomyosin, so that myosin-binding sites are exposed on the actin chain.
- The actin and myosin chains then cross-link onto one another.

...laments of myosin slide on the actin thin filaments.

...inal stage is made possible by the energy generated from the
...rolysis of adenosine.

Give some examples of smooth muscle in the body.

Examples include the inner circular and outer longitudinal muscles in the
walls of blood vessels especially arterioles, detrusor muscles of the bladder, the
myometrium of the uterus and sphincter pupillae of the iris.

How does the structure of smooth muscle differ from skeletal muscle?

There are several fundamental differences:

- Smooth muscle, as can be expected from such a wide distribution in the
  body, shows great variability in the size and morphology of the fibres –
  reflecting the variation in tasks required in different systems.
- Smooth muscle cells are often bunched into interweaving bundles of
  fibres bound together with collagen.
- Gap junctions separate individual fusiform muscle cells. This type of
  connection causes a rapid transmission of excitation throughout the
  smooth cell population in an organ, e.g. during a coordinated
  contraction wave along a segment of bowel.
- Actin and myosin filaments are not arranged as sarcomeres in smooth
  muscle. Instead, these filaments are irregularly arranged throughout
  the cell.
- The SR is more poorly developed in smooth muscle.
- T tubules are absent from smooth muscle.
- Thin (actin) filaments are bound to 'dense' bodies, which anchor them to
  the cell membrane.

How is contraction generated in smooth muscle?

- Contraction can be generated spontaneously by certain types of cell as
  their membrane potentials are unstable and decay spontaneously
  producing contraction, e.g. cardiac cells.
- Contraction may be generated by mechanical stretch of muscle fibres,
  e.g. in blood vessel walls. This is partly the basis of autoregulation of
  blood flow in cerebral, coronary and renal vessels.
- Stimulation is by neurotransmitter activation, e.g. acetylcholine-mediated
  activation of bronchial smooth muscle cell.

Note that unlike skeletal muscle, in smooth muscle, actin–myosin interaction
and subsequent contraction is mediated by the enzyme *myosin light-chain
kinase*.

Which calcium-binding protein distinguishes smooth from skeletal muscle?

- In smooth muscle, the important Ca^{2+}-binding protein is *calmodulin*. This essentially permits phosphorylation of myosin filaments.
- With skeletal muscle, the Ca^{2+}-binding protein is *troponin*, which is associated with the thin (actin) filaments.

Reflexes

What is a reflex?

A reflex is defined as an automatic response to a stimulus. It must involve a minimum of a sensor, an afferent neuron and an efferent neuron.

What are the two main types of spinal cord reflex that involve skeletal muscle activity?

Withdrawal reflex -- This is mediated by cutaneous nociceptors that connect to afferent pathways that stimulate α-motoneurons. Thus, there is automatic contraction of a muscle in response to a painful stimulus (e.g. stepping on a pin). This is a complex *polysynaptic* pathway; it also leads to inhibition of antagonistic muscle flexors (crossed reflex).

Stretch reflex -- This is the simplest reflex as it is *monosynaptic*. There is a reflex muscle contraction following stretch of fibres. It is mediated by the action of muscle spindle receptors interspersed among the regular muscle fibres. A common example is the knee-jerk reflex.

Describe the steps involved in the muscle-stretch reflex (knee jerk)

- The patellar tendon is stretched following contact with the strike of the tendon hammer. This also results in stretch of the quadriceps muscle.
- The muscle spindle fibres, which lie in parallel to the regular muscle fibres, are activated and stretched.
- The afferents arising from the spindles discharge, relaying directly back to the α-motoneuron in the ventral horn of the spinal cord.
- Thus, there is a monosynaptic pathway of connection.
- This excitatory connection leads to firing of the α-motoneuron, which leads to reflex contraction of the quadriceps.
- The spindle afferent fibres also synapse with inhibitory interneurons that inhibit the contraction of the hamstrings.

Synapses – the neuromuscular junction (NMJ)

Outline the stages of synaptic transmission

- The action potential arrives at the presynaptic neuron, which causes the opening of voltage-gated Ca^{2+} channels concentrated at the presynaptic membrane.
- There is an influx of Ca^{2+} into the presynaptic terminal, increasing the intracellular $[Ca^{2+}]$. This is the trigger for the release of transmitter into the synaptic cleft by exocytosis.
- Note that the neurotransmitter substance is stored in vesicles found at the nerve terminal. Each vesicle contains a 'quantum' of transmitter molecules.
- The neurotransmitter diffuses across the synaptic cleft, and binds onto specific receptor proteins located on the postsynaptic membrane.
- An action potential is generated in the postsynaptic cell.
- The transmitter substance is degraded, and its component parts may be recycled through uptake at the presynaptic nerve terminal.

What are the names for the changes in membrane potential caused by binding of the transmitter to the synaptic receptors?

These transient changes in the membrane potential are called 'synaptic potentials'. A transient depolarization of the postsynaptic cell is an 'excitatory postsynaptic potential' (EPSP). Similarly, a transient hyperpolarization is termed 'inhibitory postsynaptic potential' (IPSP).

What is meant by the terms 'temporal' and 'spatial' summation when referring to excitation of the postsynaptic membrane?

If the EPSP triggered by receptor binding is of sufficient magnitude, an action potential is triggered, with an influx of Na^+ or Ca^{2+}. This build-up of EPSPs at the postsynaptic membrane is called 'summation'. It may occur through two mechanisms:

Temporal summation	A rapid train of impulses from a single presynaptic cell causes EPSPs to add up, triggering an action potential in the postsynaptic cell.
Spatial summation	Multiple presynaptic neurons stimulate the postsynaptic cell simultaneously, leading to an accumulation of EPSPs, thus triggering an action potential.

What is 'synaptic facilitation'?

This is where repeated stimulation of the presynaptic neuron causes a progressive rise in the amplitude of the postsynaptic response. It arises from a local accumulation of Ca^{2+} at the presynaptic terminal and is an example of short-term synaptic plasticity.

How many NMJs may a skeletal muscle fibre have?

Despite its long length, each skeletal muscle fibre has only one neuron committed to it. Thus, there is only one NMJ per fibre.

What is the neurotransmitter at the NMJ, and what is the source of this chemical?

Acetylcholine (ACh). Intracellular choline combines with the acetyl group of acetyl coenzyme A. The catalyst for this reaction is the cytosolic enzyme choline acetyl transferase (CAT).

How is this chemical removed from the NMJ following release into the synaptic cleft?

Following unbinding from postsynaptic cholinoceptors, ACh undergoes hydrolysis into acetate and choline. This degradation is catalyzed by the enzyme acetyl cholinesterase (AChE). Choline is then recycled back into the presynaptic terminal for further Ach production.

Generally speaking, how may the cholinergic receptors be classified?

Cholinergic receptors may be *nicotinic* or *muscarinic*.

What is their distribution in the body?

Nicotinic -- Found at the NMJ, autonomic nervous system (ANS) ganglia, and at various points in the central nervous system (CNS). They are connected directly to ion channels for rapid cellular activation.

Muscarinic -- Found at postganglionic parasympathetic synapses (e.g. heart, smooth muscles and glandular tissue), in the CNS and gastric parietal cells. They are G-protein coupled, leading to either activation of K^+-channels or inhibition of adenylate cyclase.

Venous pressure

Draw the waveform of the central venous pressure (CVP), labelling the various deflections

See Figure 1.6.

What do the individual deflections represent?

a wave	Atrial contraction.
x wave	Follows the end of atrial systole.
c wave	Produced by bulging of the tricuspid valve into the atrium at the start of ventricular systole.

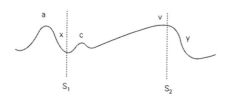

Figure 1.6 Jugular venous pressure waveform in relation to the first (S_1) and second (S_2) heart sounds.

v **wave**   Occurs due to progressive venous return to the atrium. It indicates the timing of ventricular systole, but is not directly caused by it.

y **descent**   Occurs following opening of the tricuspid valve.

Why are the veins considered the main (capacitance) vessels of the body?

The body's veins and venules are thin-walled and voluminous, and thus are capable of accommodating much of the circulating blood volume. In fact, about two-thirds of the blood volume is to be found in the venous system.

What is the normal range for the CVP?

0–10 mmHg.

Which factors determine the venous return to the heart, and hence the CVP?

Circulating blood volume	It follows that the greater blood volume, the greater the venous pressure.
Venous tone	Sympathetic stimulation in various peripheral and visceral venous beds causes venoconstriction, leading to increased venous return and venous pressure. This is an important compensatory mechanism in hypovolaemia and maintains the stroke volume and cardiac output.
Posture	Supine posture or leg elevation increases venous return.
Skeletal muscle pump	The calf pump system is particularly important in increasing the venous return during exercise, when muscle contraction compresses the deep soleus plexus of veins.
Respiratory cycle and intrathoracic pressure	During inspiration, the intrathoracic pressure falls (i.e. becomes more negative), increasing the venous return gradient to the heart. The opposite occurs during expiration.

Critical care

Agitation and sedation

Give some causes of acute confusion in the postoperative patient

- Pain, anxiety and disorientation can all commonly occur in patients in intensive care.
- Sepsis: systemic infection, or localized to chest, urinary tract, wound, etc.
- Hypoglycaemia, or hyperglycaemia with ketoacidosis.
- Respiratory failure, leading to hypoxaemia or hypercarbia: precipitating causes apart from chest infection include acute pulmonary oedema, pneumothorax, pulmonary embolism and sputum retention or atelectasis.
- Hypotension of any cause: e.g. bleeding, myocardial infarction, or arrhythmia leading to reduced cerebral perfusion.
- Acute renal or hepatic failure.
- Electrolyte disturbance: most commonly hypo- or hypernatraemia.
- Water imbalance: both dehydration and fluid overload.
- Acute urinary retention, especially in the elderly.
- Drugs: opiate analgesia, excess sedative drugs, anticholinergics.

Which investigations should you perform?

A full history and examination must be carried out so that the most pertinent investigations are performed. These investigations include:

- Arterial blood gas analysis: this determines the base excess and respiratory function,
- Serum glucose,
- Full blood cell count,
- Serum electrolytes: sodium, potassium, calcium, phosphate, magnesium, lactate (strictly speaking, a metabolite), urea and creatinine,
- Liver function tests,

- Sepsis screen: blood cultures, wound swab, urine and sputum cultures,
- Radiology, such as a chest radiograph,
- Electrocardiogram (ECG), for arrhythmias and myocardial infarction.

What is the purpose of sedation in the critical care setting?

- Anxiolysis,
- Analgesia,
- Amnesia,
- Hypnosis.

Thus, there is a reduction in the level of consciousness, but with retention of verbal communication. There is much variability on which permutation of these effects individual agents produce.

Therefore, from a practical perspective in the intensive care setting, sedative agents are used to permit tolerance of endotracheal tubes, suctioning and other bedside procedures.

How is the level of sedation determined?

There are a number of techniques in routine clinical use to determine the level of sedation attained. The most commonly employed of these is the Ramsay scoring system, which describes six levels of sedation:

Level 1 The patient is anxious and agitated or restless or both,
Level 2 The patient is co-operative, orientated and tranquil,
Level 3 The patient responds to commands only,
Level 4 Asleep. Brisk response to glabellar tap or loud auditory stimulus.
Level 5 Asleep. Sluggish response to glabellar tap or loud auditory stimulus.
Level 6 Asleep. No response to glabellar tap or loud auditory stimulus.

The ideally sedated patient attains levels 2–4.

Which classes of drug may be used?

The most commonly used classes of drug are:

Benzodiazepines	Such as diazepam and midazolam.
Intravenous (IV) anaesthetic agents	Such as propofol and ketamine.
Inhalational anaesthetic	Nitrous oxide (70%).
Opiate analgesics	Morphine and the synthetic opioids pethidine and fentanyl are popular choices. They may be combined effectively with benzodiazepines.

Trichloroethanol derivatives	Such as chloral hydrate.
Butyrophenones	Such as haloperidol. As a group, they are neurotransmitter-blocking drugs.
Phenothiazines	Such as chlorpromazine. They also act on neurotransmitter receptors.

Which of these are the most commonly used for sedation in critical care?

The most commonly used sedative drugs are propofol, benzodiazepines and the opioid analgesics.

What is the major physiological side effect of propofol?

The important side effect of propofol is hypotension on induction, which is caused by a fall in the systemic vascular resistance or myocardial depression. As with many of the other sedatives, it also leads to respiratory depression.

Burns

How common are burn injuries in the UK?

In the UK, burns account for 10 000 hospital admissions and 600 deaths per annum.

What types of burn are there?

Burns may be:

- Thermal, due to extreme heat or cold (contact, inhalational, radiation),
- Electrical,
- Chemical burns due to caustic substances (acidic or alkaline).

What criteria may be used for the assessment of thermal burns?

Burns are assessed by their extent on the body and their depth of skin penetration.

Extent -- Described in terms of the percentage (%) body surface area covered. As a rule of thumb, the area covered by the patient's palm is equivalent to 1%. Also by the 'rule of nines': anterior and posterior trunk = 18%, head and arms = 9%, legs = 18% and genitalia = 1%.

Depth -- May be superficial, partial or full-thickness: clinical determinants of the depth are:

- Presence of erythema: seen in superficial burns,
- Blisters,
- Texture: leathery skin seen with full-thickness burns,
- Sensation: burns are painful in area where there is no full-thickness penetration.

Why are burns patients susceptible to respiratory complications?

- There may be a thermal injury to the nose or oropharynx with upper airway oedema,
- Smoke inhalation can lead to hypoxia with pulmonary oedema from acute respiratory distress syndrome (ARDS),
- Inhalation of carbon monoxide,
- Inhalation of other toxic gases, such as cyanide, or the oxides of sulphur and nitrogen,
- Circumferential burns of the chest may restrict respiration,
- Aggressive fluid resuscitation may produce pulmonary oedema,
- A superadded chest infection may complicate pulmonary oedema.

Why is carbon monoxide toxic?

- It has an affinity for haemoglobin (forming carboxyhaemoglobin) about 250 times greater than that of oxygen.
- Consequently, the oxygen dissociation curve is shifted to the *left*, with poorer oxygenation of the tissues.
- It also binds to some of the respiratory chain enzymes, such as cytochrome oxidase, therefore, affecting oxygen utilization at the cellular level.

When would you suspect an impending respiratory problem?

- Fire in a confined space,
- Soot at the mouth or in the sputum,
- Burns on the face, singing of the eyebrows,
- Hoarse voice,
- Serum carboxyhaemoglobin of $>10\%$.

Why are burns patients susceptible to renal failure?

- Hypovolaemia from plasma loss reduces the renal perfusion with the development of acute tubular necrosis.
- Circulating myoglobin produces rhabdomyolysis, resulting in tubular injury and acute tubular necrosis.
- Renal failure may occur as a complication of sepsis and the systemic inflammatory response.

What are the other systemic complications of severe burns?

Aside from respiratory and renal failure, the other systemic complications are:

- 'Burns shock': hypovolaemic shock due to plasma loss following loss of skin cover. Leads to hypotension, tachycardia, increased systemic vascular resistance and a fall in the cardiac output.
- Electrolyte disturbances: hypo- or hypernatraemia, hyperkalaemia, hypercalcaemia.
- Hypothermia following loss of skin cover – convection heaters may be used.
- Systemic inflammatory response syndrome (SIRS) that can lead to multi-organ dysfunction and high mortality.
- Generalized sepsis from organisms, including gram positive (*Staphylococcus aureus*) and gram negative (*Acinetobacter* and *Pseudomonas*). The features indicating sepsis may be indistinguishable from other causes of SIRS.
- Gastric ulceration as part of the stress response.
- Coagulopathy due to disseminated intravascular coagulation and hypothermia.
- Haemolysis leading to haemoglobinuria and anaemia.

Describe the principles behind the early management of burns

Immediate and early management of burns involves adherence to the Adult Trauma Life Support (ATLS) system, involving identification of any other injuries:

- Airway and breathing: looking for the presence of respiratory distress, which may not be in evidence initially. High flow oxygen is given. May require early intubation and ventilation.
- Circulation: monitoring of fluid therapy and cardiovascular function necessitates the insertion of a central venous catheter. Arterial pressure is supported with fluids.
- Renal support involves the maintenance of the renal perfusion pressure with IV fluids. Given the added risk of rhabdomyolysis, a urinary catheter should be inserted, and the urine output maintained >1 ml/(kg h).
- Analgesia: using IV opioids or inhaled 70% nitrous oxide.
- Prevention of hypothermia with convection heaters and a warm ambient temperature. This also helps to control the hypermetabolic state.
- Stress ulcer prophylaxis is commenced.
- Prophylactic antibiotic use is controversial, and should only be used for proven sepsis.
- Surgery has a role in the emergency management of constricting circumferential thoracic eschars, which can cause respiratory embarrassment.
- Nutritional supplementation (preferably by the enteral route) should be commenced at an early stage.

How much fluid would you give?

A number of formulae to determine the rate and level of fluid replacement are available. However, ultimately, the amount of fluid given depends on the clinical situation.

- IV fluids are commenced if >15% adult or >10% paediatric burns.
- Deeper and more extensive burns may require a blood transfusion, especially in the context of other injuries.
- The ATLS guideline is 2–4 ml/kg per 1% burn in the first 24 h, half of which is to be given in the first 8 h.
- The Mount Vernon formula divides fluid administration into a number of discrete time periods. The amount of fluid given in each period is the product of the weight and the percentage of burn divided by two. The first 36 h is divided into periods of 4, 4, 4, 6, 6, and 12 h.
- Crystalloid or colloid may be used. Neither has a proven survival benefit over the other.

How do you assess the adequacy of fluid therapy?

A number of clinical parameters may be used:

- Clinical measures of the cardiac index: peripheral warmth, capillary refill time and urine output.
- Core temperature.
- Haematocrit, determined by plasma volume and red blood cell mass. This measure is unreliable if there has been a recent transfusion or haemolysis.
- Central venous pressure and its response to fluid challenges.

What are the parameters used to monitor fluid therapy?

- Skin colour,
- Heart rate,
- Blood pressure,
- Hourly urine output,
- Peripheral circulation,
- Core temperature,
- Haematocrit levels.

When is skin grafting needed?

- Deep or full thickness burns – determined at the day of burn – will not regenerate and will therefore need skin grafting. This is usually done by excision of tissue until bleeding healthy tissue is reached and then grafting.

- Deep dermal burns can either be managed in a similar way to full thickness burns or they can be left to reveal areas that might heal or regenerate, and thus only excise and graft unhealed areas.
- Superficial dermal burns are usually able to heal by regeneration from undamaged keratinocytes within 10 to 14 days. They do not require skin grafting and they usually heal with minimal scarring.
- Superficial burns heal rapidly from the remaining basal cells and re-epithelialize with minimal or no scarring. Discolouration is common in darker skin colours.

Coagulation defects

What are the basic components to normal haemostatic function?

Normal haemostatic function depends on the normal interplay of a number of components:

- Normal vascular endothelial function and tissue integrity,
- Normal platelet number and function,
- Normal amounts of the coagulation factors and their normal function,
- Presence of various essential agents, such as vitamin K and calcium,
- Balanced relationship between the fibrinolytic pathway and the clotting cascade.

What do platelets do, and what is their origin?

Platelets have a number of functions during the haemostatic response:

Vasoconstriction	During the platelet release reaction, vasoactive mediators such as serotonin, thromboxane A_2 and ADP are released.
Factor-binding	Platelet membrane phospholipids, through a reaction involving calcium and vitamin K, bind to factors II, VII, IX and X. This serves to concentrate and coordinate factors in the same area, for maximum activation.
Formation of the primary haemostatic plug	Further stabilized by platelet granule enzymes.

Platelets are formed in the bone marrow and released by megakaryocyte fragmentation.

What is von Willebrand's factor?

Von Willebrand's factor is a molecule synthesized by megakaryocytes and endothelial cells. It facilitates the binding of platelets to the subendothelial connective tissue, and binds to factor VIII.

What is the function of vitamin K?

Vitamin K, a fat-soluble vitamin, is involved in the pathway that leads to factors II, VII, IX and X binding to the surface of platelets. Specifically, it is involved in the carboxylation of these factors, allowing them to bind to calcium, and hence the surface of platelets.

Which factors are involved in the intrinsic pathway?

The factors and co-factors of the intrinsic pathway are VIII, IX, X, XI and XII.

Which factors are involved in the extrinsic pathway?

The factors and co-factors of the extrinsic pathway are tissue factor, factors VII and X.

What is the end result of the coagulation cascade?

The end product of the coagulation cascade is the formation of a stable meshwork of cross-linked fibrin around the primary platelet plug. This therefore forms the stable haemostatic plug.

Give some reasons why a surgical patient may develop a coagulopathy

Causes of a coagulopathy in the surgical patient include:

Hypothermia –– A cold patient has dysfunctioning platelets.

Massive blood transfusion –– Packed red cells do not contain platelets, so a large transfusion leads to a dilutional loss. Also, stored blood rapidly loses the function of the labile factors V and VIII.

Aspirin therapy –– Those with cardiovascular disease may be on aspirin prior to surgery. This leads to reduced platelet function by interfering with thromboxane A_2 synthesis.

Heparin therapy –– This not only interferes directly with clotting, but leads to thrombocytopenia through an immunologic mechanism – the so-called 'heparin-induced thrombocytopenia syndrome' or 'HITS'.

Dextran infusions –– These also affect platelet and coagulation factor function.

Sepsis –– A cause of DIC.

Development of postoperative acute renal or liver failure.

How may a coagulopathy be recognized in the surgical patient?

- Persisting small vessel bleeding intra-operatively, despite achieving adequate surgical haemostasis,
- Postoperative bleeding: excess blood loss from the drains,

- Platelet problems presenting as a new-onset purpuric rash,
- Bleeding from unusual areas: venepuncture or cannulation sites, epistaxis, haematuria from uncomplicated bladder catheterization.

Which tests are used to investigate coagulopathies?

- The platelet count,
- Tests of platelet function:
  - Bleeding time (range 3–8 min),
  - Adhesion studies: e.g., with epinephrine, collagen or ristocetin.
- Prothrombin time (PT): (9–15 s): a measure of the extrinsic and common pathways and the degree of warfarinization,
- Activated partial thromboplastin time (APTT): (30–40 s): a measure of the intrinsic and common pathways, and also of heparin therapy,
- Thrombin time (TT): (14–16 s): a measure of the final common pathway,
- Individual factor assay,
- Fibrin-degradation products: when testing for DIC.

Decubitus ulcers

What causes decubitus ulcers?

These result from ischaemic necrosis following continuous pressure on an area of skin. This pressure leads to restriction of the microcirculation of the area, decreased viability and ulceration.

Who are the most vulnerable to decubitus ulcers and what are the risk factors?

Bedridden patients, who are not continuously turned to relieve pressure-dependent areas, are the most vulnerable. Areas where bony prominences are present or there is a lack of fat (especially in malnourished cachectic patients) have an increased likelihood of developing these ulcers.

Immobilization, decreased cutaneous sensation and incontinence causing maceration to the skin all increase risk of ulceration.

What are the grades of ulcer (degree of damage)?

Grade I   Persistent erythema,

Grade II   Marked ulceration,

Grade III   Involvement and destruction of the subcutaneous tissue including fat and muscle.

What is the usual mode of treatment?

Prevention is best: this includes regular turning of patient who are immobile or bedridden and the use of air mattresses that can distribute pressure.

Surgical debridement of an ulcer might be needed in high-grade ulcers, while low-grade ulcers can be treated using regular wound care and dressings.

What are the other types of ulcer that can be found in the lower limb?

Venous stasis ulcers –– These are usually present around the medial and lateral malleolus, and in association with lower limb oedema. Treatment is commonly with elevation and compression stockings.

Arterial insufficiency ulcers –– These ulcers are more commonly found around the heel and the distal end of the toes. They are typically painful and need a vascular work-up.

Neuropathic ulcers –– These ulcers are found on the sole of the foot and toes. They originate at pressure points and are common in diabetic patients. They are usually painless, in contrast to arterial ulcers.

Initial evaluation of the multi-trauma patient

What worldwide system is used in assessing the multi-trauma adult patient?
Adult Trauma Life Support (ATLS).

What is it designed for?
To identify life-threatening injuries and initiate stabilizing treatment in a rapid and efficient manner, within the framework of a team.

What is the primary survey?
ABCDE:

Airway and C-spine control –– Determine the ability of air to pass unobstructed into the lungs. If patient is talking, then it is safe to assume that the airway is spontaneously maintained.

Breathing –– Determine the ability of the patient to ventilate and oxygenate. Assess the presence of bilateral air entry and monitor the oxygen saturation.

Circulation –– Establish the presence of a pulse rate and blood pressure. Identify hypovolaemia, cardiac tamponade and external sources of haemorrhage. Insert two large-bore peripheral IV cannulae, and initiate an infusion of a crystalloid, take blood samples (including arterial blood gas and glucose measurements). Control any external haemorrhaging with external pressure.

Disability –– Assess the patient's gross mental status and motor examination and record using the Glasgow Coma Scale (GCS). Examine the pupils and obtain an early assessment of spinal-cord injury by observing spontaneous limb and respiratory movements.

Exposure or Environment –– Completely remove patient clothing for a thorough examination and to avoid hypothermia with wet clothing or further injury from any toxic contact.

Subsequent steps in the primary survey should not be performed until after addressing life-threatening conditions in the earlier steps.

What other monitoring should be considered at this point?

Several monitoring and diagnostic tests can be carried out during the primary survey. These include:

- ECG,
- Continuous pulse oximetry,
- Blood-pressure monitoring,
- Foley urinary catheter.

What is the secondary survey?

The secondary survey follows the primary survey and initial resuscitation. It includes a head-to-toe examination to identify all injuries. A quick review of the primary survey should be carried out periodically to assess the response of the patient to the resuscitation efforts. History of the presentation should be sought from the patient or pre-hospital staff and any family members or involved personnel. Details of pre-existing conditions, regular medications, allergies and the time of the last meal should also be obtained.

NB: refer to the ATLS handbook for further detailed information

Fat embolism syndrome

What is the aetiology of fat embolism syndrome?

This can be triggered by both severe traumatic and non-traumatic critical illness.

- Long bone fractures. This is usually the cause, especially from closed femoral or tibial fractures. It is thought to be more common in closed injuries owing to the increased intramedullary pressure forcing fat molecules within the marrow into the systemic circulation.
- Major burns.
- Acute pancreatitis, possibly related to pancreatic lipase activity.
- Diabetes mellitus.
- Orthopaedic procedures, e.g. joint replacement.
- Decompression sickness.
- Cardio-pulmonary bypass.

What is the pathophysiology of how fat embolism syndrome develops?

There are two main theories:

Mechanical theory -- This states that fat droplets gain access to the circulation from the damaged vasculature at the site of the fracture. They are carried to the pulmonary vascular bed, where they enter the systemic circulation through arteriovenous shunts. Impaction of these fat emboli in terminal systemic vascular beds produces local ischaemia and tissue injury. This does not explain the non-traumatic cases of this syndrome.

Biochemical theory -- This explains the syndrome in terms of the release and activation of lipases by stress hormones, such as steroids and catecholamines. Lipase hydrolyzes circulating platelet-bound lipids into free fatty acids (FFA) and glycerol. These FFAs induce pulmonary damage and increase capillary permeability. Platelet activation also releases 5-hydroxy-tryptamine (5-HT), stimulating bronchospasm and vasospasm.

What are the clinical features of fat embolism syndrome and how do they relate to pathophysiology?

A number of clinical features suggest the syndrome has started. Ninety per cent of these establish themselves within three days of the onset of the trigger. Classically, there is a triad of cerebral signs, respiratory insufficiency and a petechial rash.

Cerebral features -- These are usually the earliest and most common clinical sign, occurring in up to 90% of those with the syndrome, mainly as encephalopathy or a distinct peripheral deficit, such as hemiparesis. It is believed that this is due to:

- Microvessel embolization of fat and platelet aggregates,
- Activated lipase damaging the lipid-rich cerebral matter.

Respiratory insufficiency -- This is seen as tachypnoea and cyanosis two or three days following the initial insult. This is due to:

- Pulmonary vascular occlusion by lipid emboli, leading to ventilation/perfusion (V/Q) mismatch and increased shunt,
- Pneumonitis due to mediator release, leading to increased capillary permeability and microatelectasis. This can lead to pulmonary oedema progressing to the syndrome of acute lung injury or ARDS,
- Superadded pneumonia.

Petechial rash -- This is usually seen within 36 hours as a purpura distributed in the area of the chest, axilla, mouth and conjunctiva. It arises as a result of:

- Direct embolization to cutaneous vessels,
- Following thrombocytopenia due to platelet consumption as part of overall pathophysiology.

A number of less common clinical features may also be seen:

Pyrexia	>38 °C,
Tachycardia	May be a sign of right ventricular strain,
Retinopathy	Following retinal artery embolization,
Renal impairment	With oliguria, lipiduria and haematuria.

Which of these features is pathognomonic?

In the right clinical setting, the presence of a petechial rash is pathognomonic of the fat embolism syndrome.

What is the role of further investigations in making the diagnosis of fat embolism syndrome?

Given the importance of clinical signs in making the diagnosis of this condition, further investigations have a limited role. They are mainly used in assessing the severity of the condition, and mapping out organ system involvement when planning a management strategy.

Arterial blood gas analysis	A V/Q mismatch, which may be severe enough to produce a type 1 respiratory failure.
Full blood count	• Decreased Hb from trauma, • Decreased platelet count, • Elevated erythrocyte sedimentation rate (ESR).
Clotting screen	• Increased fibrin-degradation products, • Increase APTT, • Increased TT.
Serum electrolytes	• Assesses renal function, • Reduced serum calcium, due to chelation by circulating lipids.
Urine	Lipiduria,
Sputum	Lipid-laden macrophages, and stains for lipid (e.g., by oil red-O).
Chest radiograph	Pulmonary infiltrates (described as a 'snow-storm' appearance) or infection,
ECG	Tachycardia and right ventricular strain (flipped-T waves in the anterior leads).

How is fat embolism syndrome managed?

Management lies, mainly, in supportive measures for the affected organ systems, and the prevention of complications, such as renal failure, pulmonary oedema and ARDS.

Respiratory support	With oxygenation. Can be administered as CPAP, or with mechanical ventilation if there are signs of ARDS.
Fluid and electrolyte balance	If too dry, it will worsen renal function and lead to acidosis; if overloaded, then there is exacerbation of pulmonary oedema.
General measure	Such as prophylaxis for deep vein thrombosis, nutritional support, control of sepsis, etc.

A number of specific treatments can also be used in an attempt to halt the progression, but these are unproven. They are based on an understanding of the pathophysiology.

IV ethanol	Reduces lipase activity.
Dextran 40	Used to reduce platelet and red cell aggregation, and expand the plasma – but can worsen renal dysfunction.
Heparin	Increases lipase activity, which can reduce circulation of lipids, but it increases lipase-induced tissue injury and exacerbate haemorrhage in the trauma patient.
Albumin solution	Binds to FFA, but can make pulmonary oedema worse, if it leaks through permeable capillaries in the lung.

Can fat embolism syndrome be prevented?

Yes, a number of prophylactic measures may be used to prevent progression to the syndrome:

Steroids	There is some evidence that early use of methylprednisolone is beneficial.
Early oxygen therapy	CPAP can be used to reduce V/Q deficit by limiting atelectasis.
Expedient fracture reduction and immobilization	Limits the lipid load onto the circulation.

What is the prognosis once fat embolism syndrome has established itself?

The mortality rate remains at 10–15%, but this partly reflects mortality from the underlying cause.

Intensive-care-unit admission criteria

What are the levels of intensity of care of hospital patients?

Care of hospital patients may be divided into four levels:

Level 0 The ward environment meets the needs of the patient,

Level 1 The ward patient requires the input of the critical care team for advice on optimization of care,

Level 2 High-dependency unit care – more detailed observation and intervention is required, often for a single failing organ system, or following major surgery,

Level 3 Intensive care for the support and management of two or more failing systems or for advanced respiratory support.

What is the purpose of the intensive care unit?

The intensive care unit provides advanced respiratory, cardiovascular and renal monitoring and support. It follows that conditions requiring support and monitoring must be thought reversible at the time of admission to the unit.

Give some criteria for admitting patients to the intensive care unit

- Advanced respiratory support is required, i.e. intubation and mechanical ventilation,
- Two or more organs need to be supported,
- The disease process is considered to be reversible,
- The wishes of the patient are not to be breached.

How does the cost of intensive care compare with ordinary ward care?

It has been estimated that intensive care is some three or four times more expensive than routine ward care.

What other departments must be found in the vicinity of the intensive care unit?

- The operating rooms,
- Imaging department,
- Accident and emergency,
- Obstetric department.

Physiology of immobilization

Which systems or areas of the body show physiological changes following prolonged immobilization?

- Musculoskeletal system,
- Cardiovascular system,
- Autonomic nervous system,
- Extracellular fluid compartment,
- Changes in overall composition of protein and fat.

What are these changes in the overall body composition?

Reduction in the lean body mass	This is seen as an increase in the excretion of nitrogen after the fifth day of bed-rest. The level of protein catabolism falls after several weeks, but is still higher than normal.
Increase in adipose tissue deposition	This is to replace the loss of muscle mass.
Increase in potassium excretion	Potassium is the major intracellular cation, and especially rich in muscle: its loss is an indicator of loss of total body lean tissue mass.

How long after continued bed-rest are cardiovascular changes observed?

Around three weeks of immobilization.

What are these changes?

Increase in heart rate	After three weeks, the rate increases about half a beat per minute per day of immobilization.
Reduction of stroke volume	This is associated with a measure of cardiac atrophy.
Cardiac output (CO) and arterial pressure are maintained	A result of the above antagonizing changes.
Adaptations to postural changes are impaired	This is because of impairment of inotropic and cardiac output response to a fall in arterial pressure, despite an exaggerated peripheral vascular response. The overall ANS activity is reduced, blunting cardiovascular response.

What happens to the musculoskeletal system following three weeks of bed-rest or during space flight?

Demineralization of bone -- Bone resorption exceeds bone formation and disuse osteoporosis develops. This especially occurs in load-bearing bones, such as the calcaneum. Although plasma calcium levels are not markedly elevated, large amounts of calcium are excreted in urine. Plasma concentrations of parathyroid hormones and 1,25-dihydroxycholecalciferol fall.

Muscular changes -- Reduction of muscle bulk and power (lower limbs > upper limbs).

What happens to blood volume during immobilization?

After three weeks, there may be a fall of up to 600 ml. This is due to loss of plasma volume, with a minimal fall in circulating red cell volume. This also relates to the impairment in the cardiovascular adaptation of the body to postural changes.

What are the other major risks of prolonged bed-rest?

Increased risk of deep vein thrombosis	This forms one the tenets of Virchow's triad (stasis).
Increased risk of decubitus ulcers	Mostly seen over bony prominences and the sacrum. Risk is increased in individuals who are unable to change position, such as those with spinal injuries.

Rhabdomyolysis

What is myoglobin composed of and what is its function?

Myoglobin is a respiratory pigment that is found in cardiac and skeletal muscle. It is composed of a single globin chain and a single haem component. It acts as a ready source of oxygen for muscle during times of increased activity.

How does the oxygen dissociation curve for myoglobin differ from that of haemoglobin?

The shape of the dissociation curve is hyperbolic, as opposed to sigmoidal for haemoglobin. Unlike haemoglobin, CO_2 or pH does not affect the curve.

What accounts for this difference?

The shape of the haemoglobin curve is a function of the interaction among the multiple globin chains and haem molecules. Myoglobin consists of only one globin chain and one haem molecule, so does not exhibit these interactions.

What is rhabdomyolysis?

Rhabdomyolysis is a clinical syndrome caused by the release of potentially toxic muscle cell components into the circulation. It has many triggers, including trauma, drugs, metabolic and congenital conditions.

What kind of trauma to muscle cell integrity can trigger rhabdomyolysis?

- Blunt trauma, e.g. crush injury,
- Prolonged immobilization on a hard surface, e.g. following a neck of femur fracture in the elderly,
- Massive burns,

- Strenuous and prolonged spontaneous exercise,
- Hypothermia,
- Hyperthermia or hyperpyrexia,
- Acute ischaemia and reperfusion injury.

What are the complications of rhabdomyolysis?

Acute renal failure	Develops in up to 30% of patients and thought to result from ischaemic tubular injury caused by myoglobin in the renal tubules.
Disseminated intravascular coagulation	Due to pathological activation of the coagulation cascade by the released muscle compounds.
Compartment syndrome	Muscle injury associated with a rise in compartment pressure can lead to muscle ischaemia.
Hypovolaemia	Due to haemorrhage into the necrotic muscle. This may be exacerbate the diminished renal function.
Electrolyte imbalance	Hyperkalaemia and hyperphosphataemia

What are the associated electrolyte imbalances?

- Hyperkalaemia with metabolic acidosis,
- Hypocalcaemia,
- Hyperphosphataemia,
- Hyperuricaemia.

How do you confirm the diagnosis of rhabdomyolysis?

- Elevated creatine kinase (CK), of up to five times the normal limit. Elevated CK-MM is specific to skeletal muscle injury.
- Elevated lactate dehydrogenase.
- Elevated creatinine (Cr).
- Dark urine, indicating myoglobin in urine.
- Myoglobinuria: suggested by positive dipstick to blood in the absence of haemoglobinuria.

What are the principles of management of a patient who has developed rhabdomyolysis following trauma?

The principle is largely supportive therapy.

Good hydration	To support urine output with IV crystalloid. Diuretics, such as mannitol, have been proposed to assist in this.

| **Alkalinizing agent** | Sodium bicarbonate infusion has been used to limit myoglobin-induced tubular injury in the presence of acidic urine. |
| **Management of electrolyte imbalances** | Particularly hyperkalaemia caused by release of potassium by the injured muscle and exacerbated by metabolic acidosis. In the face of worsening renal function, dialysis or haemofiltration must be considered. |

Spinal anaesthesia

What are the features of a general anaesthetic?

A general anaesthetic (GA) involves muscle relaxation, loss of consciousness (this is reversible) and a block of painful stimuli.

What is the difference between a spinal, an epidural and a regional nerve block?

- A spinal anaesthetic involves inserting a spinal needle into the subarachnoid space and injecting a combination of local anaesthetic and analgesia into the spinal canal. This will provide the required effect below the level of injection. This is commonly used in orthopaedic surgery.
- Epidural anaesthesia is similar to spinal anaesthesia except that a catheter is inserted into the epidural space (the space prior to the subarachnoid space). The catheter can remain *in situ*, providing an infusion of anaesthesia and analgesia for postoperative pain management.
- A regional nerve block targets a specific territory, such as the brachial plexus in upper limb surgery.

Which patients are suited for spinal anaesthesia?

Spinal anaesthesia is best suited for older patients and those with systemic disease, such as respiratory, cardiac, endocrine or hepatorenal disease. Many patients with mild cardiac disease benefit from the vasodilation that accompanies spinal anaesthesia. It is suitable for managing patients with trauma if they have been adequately resuscitated and are not hypovolaemic.

What are the main advantages of spinal anaesthesia?

Cost, patient satisfaction, patent airway, fewer adverse effects in patients with respiratory disease and diabetic patients, muscle relaxation of limbs, less blood loss (vs. GA) and reduced incidence of thrombosis (deep vein thrombosis and pulmonary embolism).

What are the contraindications to spinal anaesthesia?

- Clotting disorders and patients on antiplatelet (relative contraindication) or warfarin: haematoma can cause cord compression.
- Hypovolaemia: patient will become hypotensive,

- Septicaemia: increases risk of developing an epidural abscess or introducing bacteria into the intrathecal space.
- Anatomical spinal deformities (relative contraindication),
- Some neurological diseases and raised intracranial hypertension, which could cause coning.

What is the relevant anatomy in performing a spinal anaesthetic?

The spinal cord ends at L2 in adults (L3 in children). Dural puncture above this level is associated with a higher risk of spinal cord injury. The top of the iliac crests provide an anatomical landmark, indicating the level of L4/L5. The structures that will be pierced during a spinal anaesthetic are shown in Figure 2.1.

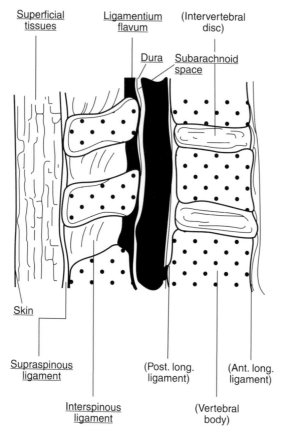

Figure 2.1
Structures that are pierced in a spinal anaesthetic (underlined).

- Skin,
- Subcutaneous fat (variable thickness),
- Supraspinous ligament (connecting the tips of the spinous processes),
- Interspinous ligament,
- Ligamentum flavum (elastic tissue running from lamina to lamina, overlying the epidural space beneath which contains fat and blood vessels; has a thick feel to it, producing a 'give' upon piercing),
- Dura,
- Subarachnoid space (which contains the spinal cord and nerve roots surrounded by CSF).

What is the cause of hypotension in spinal anaesthesia and what is the most common agent for treatment?

Hypotension occurs in spinal anaesthesia due to vasodilation from the blockage of the autonomic fibres, and the decrease in effective circulating volume. The aim of treatment is to reverse the vasodilation. The most common vasopressor (vasoconstrictor) used is ephedrine. The dose should be titrated with the blood pressure. It causes peripheral vascular constriction and increases cardiac output by increasing the heart rate and the force of myocardial contractility.

How do you assess the block?

The patient's loss of temperature sensation is tested using a cold spray, by comparing the lower limb with the arm or chest. The patient can also be asked to lift the leg; if this is not possible then the block is around the mid-lumbar region. Pain can also be tested using a sharp instrument (e.g. toothed forceps; needle puncture should be avoided). Note that the patient will feel pressure and touch, but the key is not feeling pain.

Spinal injury

What is the incidence of spinal injuries in the UK?

Three neurological syndromes are associated with incomplete cord injuries (Figure 2.2):

Central cord syndrome	Tends to occur in older individuals following hyperextension of the C-spine and compression of the cord against degenerative discs. Cord damage is centrally located.
Anterior spinal cord syndrome	The anterior aspect of the cord is injured, sparing the dorsal columns.
Brown-Séquard syndrome	Following spinal hemisection.

Central cord syndrome

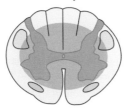

Anterior cord syndrome

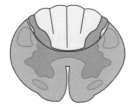

Brown-Séquard syndrome

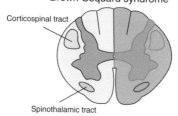

Corticospinal tract

Spinothalamic tract

Figure 2.2 Incomplete lesions of the spinal cord.

What are the patterns of deficit seen in each of the three syndromes?

Central cord syndrome –– Motor weakness affects mainly the upper limbs. Sensory loss is usually less severe.

Anterior spinal cord syndrome –– There is loss of motor function. There is also loss of pain and temperature sensation, but light touch, proprioception and vibration sense are unaffected, owing to preservation of the dorsal columns.

Brown-Séquard syndrome –– There is a motor loss below the lesion, with contralateral loss of pain and temperature sensation. There is ipsilateral loss of dorsal column function.

What deficits are seen in cases of complete injury?

The following deficits occur:

Motor deficit	Initial flaccid paralysis below the level of the lesion gives way to a spastic paralysis with increased tone and deep tendon reflexes due to loss of upper motoneuron input into the cord.
Sensory deficit	Affecting the anterolateral and posterior columns. These therefore affect the somatic and visceral components of sensation.
Autonomic deficit	Affecting the sympathetic and parasympathetic outputs of the cord.

When would you suspect a spinal trauma in an unconscious trauma patient?

- Presence of multiple trauma, especially with head injuries.
- Priapism in the male.
- Paradoxical respiration due to diaphragmatic breathing when there is paralysis of the intercostal muscles. The level of the lesion in these cases is between C5 and C8.
- Positive Babinski's reflex following loss of the upper motoneuron input. However, this is unreliable.

Why may the trauma patient with a spinal injury exhibit bradycardia?

- Loss of sympathetic outflow from the damaged cord,
- Following a reflex increase in the cranial parasympathetic outflow due to airway suctioning,
- The Cushing reflex due to elevated intracranial pressure if there is an associated head injury,
- Pre-existing bradycardia due to cardiac disease or the use of drugs, such as β-adrenoceptor blockers.

Why may spinal cord lesions lead to hypotension?

- Loss of sympathetic outflow: there is loss of vasomotor tone leading to reduced systemic vascular resistance and, therefore, reduced arterial pressure.
- Loss of sympathetic outflow can also produce bradycardia, which leads to a fall in the cardiac output and reduced arterial pressure.
- Occult blood loss, e.g. following blunt abdominal trauma with a visceral or vascular injury. Haemorrhage may be missed – it is easy to ascribe hypotension to the spinal injury alone.

What are the dangers of autonomic dysfunction in these situations?

- Occult blood loss may be missed if there is hypotension, being erroneously ascribed to spinal trauma.
- This may lead to overhydration during fluid resuscitation, leading to pulmonary oedema.
- Hypotension reduces the cerebral perfusion pressure in the face of a head injury and rising intracranial pressure.
- Bradycardia may be exacerbated when carrying out manoeuvres that stimulate the cranial parasympathetic outflow, e.g. intubation, airway suction, bladder distension. This may induce cardiac arrest. IV atropine must be at hand to reverse this process.
- May lead to hypothermia due to loss of vasomotor control.

What is 'spinal shock'?

This is a temporary state of flaccid paralysis that usually occurs very soon after a spinal injury, and may take three or four weeks to resolve. This is caused by the loss of excitatory stimuli from supraspinal levels.

What drug has been used to minimize the extent of spinal injury following trauma?

High dose IV methylprednisolone has been used to limit secondary spinal injury from free radicals produced following trauma. For the most beneficial effect, it must be given within eight hours of trauma. This remains controversial, with no strong evidence supporting it, and it is thus no longer commonly used.

What does the immediate management of spinal injuries entail?

Immediate management involves prevention of secondary injury and management of potential complications associated with spinal injury:

- C-spine immobilization and careful handling of the patient can limit the damage if the spine has sustained an unstable injury.
- Other injuries have to be sought, e.g. abdominal trauma or pulmonary injury (which can tip the patient into respiratory failure).
- Respiratory management with supplementary oxygen. If there is a ventilatory failure, mechanical ventilation may be required.
- Management of hypotension, which starts with exclusion of haemorrhage as the cause. Judicious use of IV fluids reduces the risk of pulmonary oedema. The arterial pressure may be supported with drugs such as atropine, α-adrenoceptor agonists or the use of temporary cardiac pacing to increase the heart rate.
- Prevention of hypothermia.
- Prevention of gastric dilatation following the paralytic ileus of autonomic dysfunction. This involves nasogastric tube insertion. Gastric dilatation may splint the diaphragm, leading to respiratory failure.
- Bladder catheterization is required, owing to the risk of acute urinary retention with overflow incontinence.
- Surgical intervention may be required for unstable injuries, in the form of spinal fracture immobilization and stabilization.

What are the important issues surrounding long-term management?

The most important aspect of long-term management is rehabilitation.

- Prevention of decubitus ulcers,
- Nutritional support for high spinal injuries in the form of percutaneous enteral feeding,

- Bowel care with regular enemas and bulk-forming agents,
- Bladder care with intermittent catheterization,
- Physiotherapy to help clear lung secretions (minitracheostomy may be required) and prevent limb contractures,
- Psychological support and counselling as required.

What is the difference between a Jefferson fracture and a hangman's fracture?

Jefferson fracture –– This is a burst fracture of C1 (atlas), best seen on the peg view. It can be seen as a widening of the lateral masses and loss of congruity with the axis beneath. This is generally a stable injury.

Hangman's fracture –– A fracture of C2 (axis) caused by hyperextension of the neck with the force of the occiput and the atlas bearing down on pedicle of C2.

What is the chance of recovery from these spinal cord injuries?

The best prognosis is from a Brown-Séquard syndrome (see Figure 2.2), where recovery is more than 90%. There is a 75% chance of recovery from a central cord syndrome, and only a 10% recovery from an anterior cord syndrome.

Systemic response to trauma

Give some examples of stimuli that may activate the systemic stress response

- Trauma resulting in pain and tissue injury,
- Surgery,
- Infection: endotoxin is a powerful stimulus,
- Hypothermia,
- Severe acid–base disturbances,
- Acute hypoglycaemia.

Which four physiological systems are involved in coordinating the systemic stress response?

Sympathetic nervous system –– Producing changes in the cardiovascular, endocrine and metabolic systems, e.g. promotes hyperglycaemia and activation of the rennin-angiotensin-aldosterone (RAA) system.

Endocrine system –– Glucocorticoid release is stimulated by adrenocorticotropic hormone (ACTH) following the stress stimulus. Their plasma levels remain elevated for as long as the stimulus is present. Other hormones that are increased during the response are glucagon, thyroxine, growth hormone, histamine and endogenous opioids.

Acute phase response –– With the release of cytokines, prostaglandins, leucotrienes and kinins.

Microcirculatory system –– With changes in the vascular tone and permeability affecting tissue oxygen delivery. Vasoactive mediators, such as nitric oxide, prostaglandins and platelet-activating factor, induce vasodilatation and increase capillary permeability.

What are the main glucocorticoids in the body? Give some examples of some of their systemic effects

The two main active glucocorticoids in the body are cortisol and corticosterone. Their effects are:

Metabolic

Glucose metabolism	Stimulation of gluconeogenesis and peripheral antagonism of insulin leads to hyperglycaemia and glucose intolerance.
Protein	Increase uptake of amino acids into the liver and promotion of protein catabolism in the peripheral tissues, such as muscle.
Lipid	Stimulation of lipolysis in adipose tissue.

Mineralocorticoid activity –– Promoting sodium and water retention with loss of potassium, all being mediated at the renal level.

Other

- Anti-inflammatory, immunosuppressive and anti-allergic actions.
- Coordination of the stress response with a permissive effect on the actions of other hormones.

Draw a diagram showing the change in the basal metabolic rate following a traumatic insult to the body

See Figure 2.3.

What happens during the two phases of the metabolic response?

Ebb phase –– There is a reduction in the metabolic rate in the 24 hours following the stimulus.

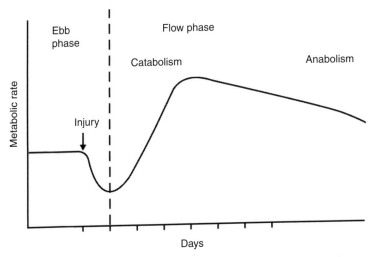

Figure 2.3 Changes in the metabolic rate following traumatic insult to the body.

Flow phase –– An increase in the metabolic rate, with generalized catabolism, negative nitrogen balance and glucose intolerance. The degree of metabolic increase depends on the type of the initiating insult.

Why is there a fall in the urine output immediately following a traumatic insult such as surgery? When does this resolve?

Following surgery, there is activation of the RAA system and increased release of antidiuretic hormone as part of the response. Thus, the urine output may remain low despite adequate volume replacement. This is usually resolved in 24 h, but sodium retention may persist for several days longer.

Why may metabolic alkalosis develop and what effect does this have on oxygen delivery to the tissues?

The mineralocorticoid effects of cortisol and aldosterone promote sodium retention at the expense of potassium. Loss of potassium can lead to metabolic alkalosis. With the reduction of H^+ that defines metabolic alkalosis, the oxygen dissociation curve is shifted to the *left* (increased oxygen affinity), reducing tissue oxygen delivery. Note that in the latter stages of the response, if there is a fall in tissue perfusion, then the patient can become acidotic.

What changes may occur in the various organ systems during the systemic stress response?

Cardiac output	Increases in the initial stages.
Lungs	Hyperventilation leads to a respiratory alkalosis. In the latter stages, as part of the systemic inflammatory response, acute lung injury and ARDS may supervene.
Liver	Reduction in the production of albumin.
Clotting	Systemic activation of the coagulation cascade, which if severe enough, can lead to disseminated intravascular coagulation (DIC).

Chapter

3

Surgical pathology

Bone tumours

Which are more common, primary bone tumours or metastatic bone tumours?

Metastatic bone tumours are the commonest tumour of the skeletal system, usually deposited in bone. They are usually of an epithelial origin, or occasionally sarcomas, and metastasize to bone.

What are the five common malignant neoplasms in bone (in order of frequency)?

- Breast: most commonly metastasize to ribs, thoracic vertebrae, clavicles,
- Prostate: reaches bone by venous spread, and is most common in the lumbosacral spine and pelvis,
- Bronchus,
- Kidney,
- Thyroid.

Arterial spread may result in deposition anywhere in the skeleton but is most common in flat bones, the vertebrae and the proximal ends of the humerus and femur.

What is the commonest malignant neoplasm *arising in* bone?

Myeloma: it originates in the haemopoietic tissue of red marrow. It is occasionally solitary but often found to be multiple. It tends to occur in patients past the fifth decade and commonly affects the pelvis and spine. It forms about half of primary malignant tumours arising in bone. The tumour cells resemble plasma cells.

What is the commonest malignant neoplasm *derived from* bone tissue?

Osteosarcoma: it arises from bone cells that are undifferentiated and capable of forming musculoskeletal tissue, such as bone, cartilage and collagenous tissue. It usually occurs under the age of 30 with a male dominance and usually in the metaphysis of long bones. A quarter of primary malignant bone tumours are osteosarcomas. Chondrosarcomas, arising from chondroblasts producing chondroid and collagen (not bone), make up 15%.

What are the effects of primary bone neoplasms on bone?

- Most tumours stimulate bone resorption, which appears as a translucent area on X-rays.
  - This could either cause the cortex to expand from the inside with bone deposition from the outside, *or*
  - It can cause a breach through the cortex into the soft tissue, causing the periosteum to be elevated from the bone, and the appearance of a triangle of new bone formation, called the Codman's triangle.
- Other tumours stimulate bone formation, which alternatively appears as a dense area on X-rays.
- Tumours of cartilage are characterized by having a spongy trabecular or honeycomb appearance.
- Bone tumours may, through their effect, weaken the bone, giving rise to pathological fractures.

What is a bone cyst and what common types are there?

A bone cyst is a non-neoplastic fluid-filled lesion that arises in bone, which has some characteristics of a tumour. These cysts usually occur in the metaphysis of long bones.

Simple or unicameral bone cyst	Fluid-filled cysts most found in the humerus, occurring in the first and second decade with a male to female ratio of 2:1. They usually present as a pathological fracture or an incidental finding on X-ray. The pathogenesis is unknown.
Aneurysmal bone cyst	Spongy blood-filled cyst-like cavity in bone, occurring in the second decade and usually painful. May be due to an arteriovenous malformation.
Subchondral bone cyst	Frequently seen in osteoarthritis as well as Paget's disease of bone.

What benign neoplasms arise in bone?

Osteoma	A hamartomatous mass from the surface of the bone with a radiodense area on X-ray. Only affects the skull.
Osteoid osteoma	A lesion causing chronic pain relieved by aspirin. X-ray appearance of a dense sclerotic area with a central translucent nidus. Can affect any bone but the skull.

Osteoblastoma	Rare primary benign neoplasm that is very similar to osteoid osteomas.
Osteoclastoma (giant cell tumour)	The origin of the osteoclasts is unknown. They affect young adults 10–20 years after epiphyseal fusion. Most common at the distal femur and proximal tibia. Expands the bone eccentrically, starting from the metaphysis going into epiphysis. 10% behave aggressively.
Osteochondroma	A solitary lesion but can be found in multiple osteochondromatosis.
Enchondroma	A hamartomatous mass of cartilage arising in the metaphysis (multiple type: Ollier's disease).
Chondroblastoma	Rare tumour affecting the epiphysis of adolescents.

Deep vein thrombosis (DVT)

What is a deep vein thrombosis?

It is a thrombus or clot formation in the large veins of the extremities or pelvis.

What is Virchow's triad?

Virchow's triad (Virchow: a pathologist of the nineteenth century) comprises: venous stasis (e.g. long-haul flights, bed-rest, incompetent venous valves); endothelial injury (e.g. any injury to the lower limb); and hypercoagulable state (e.g. in malignancy, pregnancy, use of the oral contraceptive pill). This triad portrays the risk factors that may cause a DVT.

What are the risk factors for postoperative DVT?

- History of thrombosis (deep vein thrombosis, pulmonary embolism),
- Lower limb surgery,
- Any surgery that entails or leads to immobilization,
- Active malignancy,
- Obesity,
- Oral contraceptive pill,
- Pregnancy,
- Blood disorders that would increase the viscosity of the blood.

What do patients usually present with?

Unilateral limb pain (especially along the deep veins), tense swelling, pitting oedema, erythema.

What modalities are used to aid diagnosis?

Blood tests: to rule out infection, including D-dimers (when negative can be used to rule out a deep vein thrombosis in low-risk patients). Doppler ultrasound is the radiological imaging of choice for detecting deep vein thromboses.

Gangrene

What is the definition of gangrene?

Gangrene is necrosis of tissue. It occurs when there is a loss of blood supply to that tissue due to injury or infection. Gangrene is a serious condition that can be life- or limb-threatening. Diabetes and smoking increase the risk of getting gangrene.

Where are you most likely to find gangrene?

In the lower extremities.

What are the three main types of gangrene?

Dry gangrene –– This is caused by a lack of blood supply (ischaemia), usually due to thrombosis from atherosclerosis, and commonly begins at the distal aspect of a limb, specifically the toes and feet of elderly patients. It is mainly caused by arterial occlusion. Dry gangrene spreads slowly, and the affected part becomes dry with black discolouration. Auto-amputation is characteristic if the gangrenous tissue cannot be surgically excised.

Wet gangrene –– This occurs in moist tissues and organs, secondary to bacterial infection colonizing the area. Wet gangrene has a generally poorer prognosis than dry gangrene owing to septicaemia from the accumulation of toxins released by the bacteria. Vessel occlusion is predominantly venous, in contrast to dry gangrene.

Gas gangrene –– This is caused by a bacterial exotoxin-producing clostridial species commonly found in soil and other anaerobes (usually *Clostridium perfringens*). This leads to necrosis, production of gas within the tissues and severe sepsis. There can be rapid progression to toxaemia and shock and gas gangrene should be treated as an emergency.

What is the cause of the dark discolouration in dry gangrene?

Liberation of the haemoglobin from haemolysed red blood cells. This is acted on by bacteria, resulting in the formation of iron sulphide, which is black in colour and remains in tissues.

What is the main course of treatment of established gangrene?

Surgical debridement with amputation in many cases, as the tissue is often no longer viable. Antibiotics for the treatment of infection are usually ineffective as the blood supply in the region of gangrene is poor and does not allow for drug delivery.

Gout

What is gout?

Gout was known as the 'disease of kings', owing to its association with rich foods and alcohol. It is a metabolic disease characterized by the deposition of monosodium urate (MSU) crystals in soft tissues.

Gout is caused by deposition of MSU crystals in poorly vascularized tissue, articular cartilage, ligaments, bursae and synovial membranes.

Distal joints of the hand, feet, elbows and knees are usually affected, but characteristically gout affects the metatarso-phalangeal joint (MTPS) of the great toes.

Is there a family history associated with the disease? Is there a sex preference?

- A family history is usually found in less than half of patients.
- There is male-to-female dominance of 7:1. Females with gout tend to be postmenopausal.

Are purines or pyrimidines involved in gout?

- A high level of uric acid in the body is referred to as hyperuricaemia. Purines, and not pyrimidines, are involved in hyperuricaemia. Purines, which are adenine or guanine, are metabolized in a different manner than are pyrimidines. They are degraded to hypoxanthine, which is metabolized by xanthine oxidase to xanthine then to uric acid, which is excreted in urine.
- Pyrimidines are unrelated to gout. They are metabolized into ammonium salts and urea, and not uric acid.

    Purine → hypoxanthine → xanthine (by xanthine oxidase) → uric acid = excretion in urine

How does allopurinol work?

Allopurinol is a xanthine oxidase inhibitor, which would block the metabolism of hypoxanthine to xanthine, hence its use as a maintenance drug to prevent gout.

What are the predisposing conditions of the disease?

- Common chronic diseases associated with gout are obesity, alcoholism, hypertension, hypertriglyceridaemia and ischaemic heart disease,
- High dietary intake of purines (e.g. high meat intake, alcohol consumption) – diet alone is generally not sufficient to cause hyperuricaemia,
- Decreased purine biosynthesis (lack of serum enzyme uricase),
- Medications: thiazide diuretics and antimetabolites.

Can gout and hyperuricaemia be present independent of each other?

Yes, but they usual occur mutually – a patient with hyperuricaemia is likely to develop gout.

How do you classify hyperuricaemia?

Primary	Abnormality in xanthine-hypoxanthine handling: in the event of a deficiency of phosphoribosyl transferase, xanthine and hypoxanthine cannot be recycled into purines and thus they are excreted, with an endpoint being uric acid.
Secondary	
Increased purine breakdown with increased formation of uric acid	This occurs in increased cell turnover and apoptosis (e.g. malignancy after chemotherapy or severe psoriasis).
Decreased excretion of urate	This occurs in chronic renal failure, as well as the use of various medications including thiazide diuretics.

What are the complications of gout?

Complications of gout are secondary conditions, symptoms or other conditions that are related to gout:

- Osteoarthritis due to joint destruction, immobility at time of an attack of gout, association with carpal tunnel syndrome,
- Renal calculi developing from urate accumulation – urate stones,
- Renal failure,
- Scleritis.

Heterotopic ossification

What is calcification?

It is the process in which calcium builds up in body tissue, leading to hardening of tissue: 99% of calcium entering the body is deposited in teeth and bones. Calcification can be a normal or abnormal event.

What is heterotopic ossification (HO)?

This is the presence of bone in soft tissue, where bone does not normally exist, e.g. muscle. It is seen as predominantly an acquired condition.

It is most commonly seen in post-traumatic situations (extremity fractures) or after elective orthopaedic surgery, in the presence of spinal-cord injury or neurological dysfunction. The common sites are around the hip and the elbow.

The exact cause is unknown. One theory is that mixed signals stimulate normally dormant osteoprogenitor cells, promoting bone growth. If present in soft tissue, this causes heterotopic ossification.

What treatment is available for HO?

- Bisphosphonates have been proposed, as a preventative measure for limiting further HO,
- Indomethacin (a prostaglandin synthesis inhibitor) is used to suppress mesenchymal cells, and prevent recurrence,
- Radiotherapy as a single dose has also been shown to have results around the peri-articular regions in both upper (elbow) and lower limbs, without increasing the risk of infection or bleeding.

Lymphoedema

What is a lymphoedema?

It is a disruption of the lymphatic circulation that results in peripheral oedema and possible chronic infection of the limbs.

What are the causes of lymphoedema?

It can be hereditary or congenital, e.g. Milroy's disease; or secondary to injury, e.g. surgery involving lymph node dissection. In underdeveloped countries, parasitic infection can lead to lymphatic obstruction (filariasis). It can also be caused by compromising of the lymphatic system secondary to cellulitis.

How is this condition managed?

Causes of this condition need to be identified. There is no curative treatment: management is directed at symptoms. Mobilization, exercise, massage therapy and pressure garments can all help counteract and limit fluid accumulation. Vigilance is necessary in inspecting for cellulitis with prompt gram-positive antibiotic coverage if indicated.

What similar condition should not be confused with lymphoedema?

Venous insufficiency. This condition can be confused with lymphoedema, as oedema can be present. If venous insufficiency is left untreated, it can progress into a mixed lymphatic and venous disorder.

Myeloma

What is myeloma?

- Neoplasm of bone marrow that is composed of plasma cells that result in lytic bone lesions in the red marrow and monotypic globulin in the plasma.
- It is called a plasmacytoma when proliferating plasma cells form a recognizable mass outside the marrow.

- Abnormal plasma cells can be found in various tissues.
- Usually there is multiple myeloma.

What are the signs and symptoms of myeloma?

Many organs can be affected by myeloma and clinical features vary greatly. The common tetrad of multiple myeloma is remembered with the mnemonic CRAB – elevated calcium, renal failure, anaemia and bone lesions.

Symptoms are (in descending order of incidence):

Bone pain –– Usually involves ribs and spine, and worsens with activity. A pathological fracture should be suspected if persistent localized pain is present. Vertebral fractures can lead to extradural spinal cord compression – a surgical emergency. Over-activation of osteoclasts causes bone resorption and results in lytic lesions, which are best seen on plain radiographs. They show characteristic 'punched-out' resorptive lesions, and a pepper-pot skull appearance. This process leads to release of calcium and resultant hypercalcaemia, with its complications.

Infection –– Most common infections are pneumonias (e.g., *Streptococcus pneumoniae* and *Staphylococcus aureus*) and pyelonephritis (e.g. *Escherichia coli* and other gram-negative organisms). The greatest risk period is after the start of chemotherapy. Immune deficiency ensues due to the decreased production and increased destruction of antibodies. This also results in diffuse hypogammaglobulinaemia.

Renal failure –– Both acute and chronic can occur, commonly due to hypercalcaemia. Bence-Jones proteins can also cause tubular damage. Other causes are amyloid deposition in the glomeruli, hyperuricaemia, recurrent pyelonephritis and local tumour infiltration.

Anaemia –– Usually normocytic and normochromic. This results from the replacement of normal bone marrow by infiltrating tumour cells and inhibition of haematopoiesis by cytokines.

Neurological symptoms –– Symptoms secondary to hypercalcaemia are fatigue, malaise, confusion and weakness. Hyperviscosity of the blood could result in retinopathy and visual changes. Radicular pain, loss of bowel or bladder control may occur as a result of to cord compression, while neuropathies, e.g. carpal tunnel syndrome, may result from amyloid infiltration of peripheral nerves.

Bleeding diathesis and bruising –– From binding to factor X and hyperviscosity.

What investigations would be needed to aid diagnosis?

Blood markers	Unexplained anaemia; kidney dysfunction; high ESR; high serum protein; raised calcium; protein electrophoresis (paraprotein band – monoclonal or protein M).

Urine	Bence-Jones proteins via protein electrophoresis.
Skeletal survey	Lytic lesions on X-rays of the skull, axial skeleton and proximal long bones.
MRI	More sensitive than X-rays.
Bone marrow biopsy	To determine the percentage of bone marrow occupied by plasma cells.

Osteoarthritis

What is osteoarthritis (OA)?

This is the most common form of arthritis. It is a degenerative disease of the synovial joints characterized by articular cartilage loss with an accompanying peri-articular bone response.

It is often called osteoarthrosis, as it is essentially a non-inflammatory condition.

How is osteoarthritis classified?

Primary
- Unknown aetiology,
- 15% of UK population,
- Various associations but no known cause.

Secondary (where a reason can be identified as the cause of the OA)
- Gout,
- Rheumatoid arthritis (RA),
- Paget's disease,
- Previous septic joint,
- Previous intra-articular fracture,
- Biomechanical misalignment,
- Congenital disorders, such as developmental dysplasia of the hip (DDH), Perthes' disease, achondroplasia,
- Avascular necrosis.

What joints are commonly affected?
- Hip,
- Knee,
- Shoulder,
- Vertebral column,
- Elbow,
- Interphalangeal joints of the hand,
- Foot.

What are the common symptoms of osteoarthritis?

- Pain is usually the presenting feature: night pain is usually characteristic of significant OA.
- Stiffness in the joint affecting activities of daily living. (Specifically stiffness that gets worse at the end of the day, in contrast with RA, which improves by the end of the day.)
- Altered gait.

What are the radiological changes seen on X-ray?

- Joint space narrowing,
- Subchondral cyst formation,
- Subchondral sclerosis,
- Osteophyte formation.

Osteomyelitis

What is osteomyelitis?

It is inflammation of bone and bone marrow. It is almost always caused by infection secondary to direct spread from a soft tissue infection (80%) in adults, or by haematological spread (20%), which is more common in children, seeding in the metaphyses of long bones.

What are the causes of osteomyelitis?

Infective cause is the most common cause.

- This can be due to any organism, but bacterial causes are dominant.
- Infection can be either direct or haematogenous.
- In almost 50% of cases, no organism is identified.

Non-infective causes include radiotherapy.

What are the commonest organisms?

- *Staphylococcus aureus* is responsible for around 80% of osteomyelitis,
- Others include *E. coli*, *Streptococcus*, *Pseudomonas*,
- *Salmonella* should be suspected in patients with sickle cell disease,
- Viruses,
- Fungi,
- Parasites.

What are the classical pathological sequelae of osteomyelitis?

- Acute infection, commonly at the metaphysis,
- Suppuration: pus develops in marrow cavity,

Table 3.1 Organisms associated with osteomyelitis

If	Think
Most people	*S. aureus*
IV drug user	*S. aureus* or *Pseudomonas*
Sickle cell disease	*Salmonella*
Hip or knee replacement	*Staphylococcus epidermidis*
Foot wound	*Pseudomonas*
Chronic	*S. aureus, Pseudomonas* or *Enterobacter*
Diabetes	Polymicrobial, *S. aureus, Pseudomonas, Streptococci* or anaerobes

- Sequestrum of the dead bone within the periosteum forming the inner aspect of the infected bone area,
- Involucrum: reaction of the periosteum to encompass the infected site by forming new bone,
- Cloacae: holes formed in the involucrum where pus formed discharges,
- Sinus: this is formed via the tracts created from the cloacae towards the skin,
- This can lead to septicaemia.

What X-ray findings do you expect to be seen?

- Classically, symptoms become evident 10 days after the acute onset of infection.
- 90% of X-rays would show radiological evidence of osteomyelitis at three weeks, including periosteal elevation, cortical reaction and new bone formation.
- Evidence of soft tissue swelling.

What are the late complications of osteomyelitis?

- Malignant change in the sinus – Marjolin's ulcer (squamous cell carcinoma),
- Septicaemia,
- Suppurative arthritis.

Osteoporosis

What is osteoporosis?

- It means 'porous bone' (Greek).
- It is a reduction in the bone mineral density (BMD), with a deterioration of the bone micro-architecture.
- The bone is fully mineralized, but the trabecular plates are thinned and reduced.
- This leads to bone fragility and increased risk of fracture.
- Afflicts 55% of people over the age of 50.
- One-third of women over 50 have osteoporosis.

How is it classified?

- Localized,
- Primary:
  - Menopausal (Type 1),
  - Age-related (Type 2; male to female ratio, 1:2).
- Secondary:
  - Due to chronic disease, use of medication or immobility (disuse),
  - Can occur in any age and in both males and females.

How is it defined?

- It is defined by the WHO as a bone mineral density 2.5 standard deviations or more below the mean peak of bone mass on a dual-energy absorptiometry X-ray (DEXA).
- Serum calcium, alkaline phosphatase and vitamin D levels are normal.
- X-rays show global demineralization after >1/3 of bone density is lost.

What are the commonest insufficiency fractures caused by osteoporosis?

- Proximal femoral fractures (including neck-of-femur fractures),
- Distal radius fractures,
- Vertebral compression fractures,
- Fractures can occur after minimal trauma, but are more commonly due to simple falls.

What are the risk factors for generalized osteoporosis?

- Sex: F>M: women have less bone to start, and bone resorption is more rapid after menopause,
- Body size: thin-boned women are at higher risk,

- Age: common in over 50s,
- Family history,
- Ethnic origin: more common in those of European and Asian origin,
- Nutrition: low dietary intake of calcium and vitamin D (lack of sunlight),
- Excessive intake of alcohol,
- Smoking,
- Immobility or lack of weight-bearing exercise,
- Low levels of sex hormones,
- Chronic use of steroids,
- Chronic use of heparin.

What is the aim of treatment?

The aim is to prevent bone loss and therefore prevent fractures.

What are the treatment options?

- Smoking cessation,
- Increase in weight-bearing exercises,
- Calcium and vitamin D supplementation appear to help, although the effect on fracture reduction is not clear,
- Many pharmacological agents are used but the most common are:
  - Bisphosphonates are usually considered as first-line treatment. These are antiresorptive agents that work primarily on reducing bone resorption
  - Hormone replacement therapy has been shown to decrease the rate of bone loss in postmenopausal women; however, recent studies suggest a risk of heart disease and other risks that may outweigh the benefits for the prevention of chronic conditions. This remains controversial.
  - Strontium works by suppressing the action of the osteoclasts, which break down bone, or by stimulating the action of the osteoblasts, which build bone.

Pathological fractures

What is a pathological fracture?

A fracture through abnormal or diseased bone and commonly occurring with little or no trauma.

What are some causes of pathological fractures?

- The most common cause is osteoporosis,
- Metastatic bone disease (lytic, blastic, or mixed lesions) secondary to carcinomas that metastasize to bone: breast, brain, thyroid, kidney and prostate.

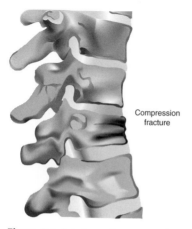

Compression fracture

Figure 3.1 Anterior wedge compression fracture of the spinal vertebra.

- Metabolic bone disease (rickets, osteomalacia),
- Osteogenesis imperfecta,
- Induced by radiotherapy (bone necrosis) or steroid use.

How do pathological osteoporotic fractures of the spine present?

Patients often complain of sudden pain and, at times, an audible 'crunch', and can present with symptoms of cord compression if there has been retropulsion of the fracture fragments into the spinal canal.

X-rays reveal compression fractures of the spinal vertebra(e), and commonly appear as a wedge or with a collapse of the entire body.

Peripheral arterial disease

What is the definition peripheral arterial disease?

This is the occlusion of the blood supply to the extremities (upper or lower limbs) by atherosclerotic plaques, potentially leading to ischaemia. It is more common to affect the lower limbs in comparison to the upper limbs.

What are the clinical manifestations of acute ischaemia?

- The clinical manifestations are dependent on the specific vessels involved, including the extent and rate of the obstruction caused and whether or not collateral vessels are present.
- The 6 Ps of ischaemia are: pain, pallor, pulselessness, paralysis, paraesthesia and poikilothermia.
- The patient usually presents with intermittent claudication, which is characterized by reproducible leg pain that occurs on exertion and is relieved at rest. Pain at rest is an indication of disease progression.
- A painful cold foot is indicative of ischaemia.

What signs would indicate aorto-iliac disease?

Buttock claudication, decreased (or absent) femoral pulses and male impotence.

What signs would indicate femoro-popliteal disease?

Calf claudication and absent pulses in the popliteal artery and the distal vessels.

What is the ankle–brachial pressure index (ABPI)?

- This is the ankle systolic blood pressure divided by the brachial systolic blood pressure.
- The normal range spans from 0.9–1.2.
- A value >1.2 indicates abnormal vessel hardening due to peripheral vessel disease (PVD).
- A value of 0.5–0.8 indicates the presence of moderate arterial disease. Mixed ulcers may be present, and claudication usually occurs when ABPI <0.6.
- A value <0.5 indicates severe arterial disease, with arterial ulcers developing and rest pain often present.
- The ABPI measurement is unreliable in patients with arterial calcification, owing to the decrease in the arterial compressibility. This is commonly present in diabetic patients.

What is the treatment of arterial disease?

- This would involve preventative measures and controlling the underlying condition, including risk factors of diabetes, hypercholesterolaemia, and other cardiac risk factors.
- Exercise promotes the development of collateral circulation.
- Medical therapy, such as aspirin and anti-coagulants can be used to prevent clot formation.
- Angioplasty and stenting might be attempted at the area of occlusion or narrowing. The alternative in evidence of acute or chronic ischaemia would be embolectomy, thrombectomy, thrombolysis or arterial bypass.
- Amputation would be required when all other forms of management fail and the limb is deemed unsalvageable.

Rheumatoid arthritis

What is rheumatoid arthritis (RA)?

This is a multisystem joint disease of unknown aetiology, occurring mostly in middle-aged people, and more commonly in women than in men.

It is an immune-mediated disease of the joints, with inflammation and destruction of the synovial surfaces. It can affect all joint types.

What happens to the joint and surrounding tissue in RA?

- Synovial inflammation followed by thickening and increased vascularity. Eventual destruction of the synovial surfaces with granulation tissue around the damaged areas.

- Infiltration of vascular synovium at the periphery of the articular cartilage, leading to cartilage destruction.
- Bone erosion, subchondral cysts, local bone osteopenia and, possibly, ankylosis.
- Significant damage to joint capsule.

How does it usually present?

- Slowly increasing stiffness and aches in the joints; may progress into joint deformity and significant disability.
- May start with one joint and progress to others in a variable manner and timeframe.

Are tendons affected by RA?

- Yes, a similar inflammatory process can occur in the tendons.
- This is most commonly seen in tendons of the hand, with residual flexion–extension deformities (Boutonniere and swan-neck deformities), ulnar deviation of the fingers, Z-deformity of the thumb, and radial deviation of the wrist.
- Spontaneous ruptures of the tendons can occur.

What are the extra-articular manifestations of RA?

- Rheumatoid nodules (common in one in three RA patients),
- Rheumatoid vasculitis,
- Pericarditis,
- Pleurisy,
- Scleritis,
- Amyloid deposition,
- Tophi deposition.

What is the natural history of the condition?

- It is a progressive condition.
- Remission can occur but is usually temporary. Occasionally the disease can burn out.
- Deformities are permanent and often need surgical correction.
- Secondary osteoarthritic changes are very common.

Sarcoma

What is a sarcoma?

A malignant tumour composed of connective tissue cells (the name indicates what the tumour is made of). It can arise from any tissue within the body. Half of all sarcomas occur in the musculoskeletal system. They tend to metastasize via the blood stream – haematogenous spread.

What is the difference between a sarcoma and a carcinoma?

A carcinoma is also a malignant tumour, but it is composed of epithelial cells.

Name some musculoskeletal sarcomas

Osteosarcoma	Arises from bone cells that are undifferentiated and capable of forming musculoskeletal tissue, such as bone, cartilage and collagenous tissue. It usually occurs under the age of 30 with a male dominance and usually in the metaphysis of long bones (50% femur). The tumour grows rapidly, and pain is the dominant feature – commonly waking the patient at night. A quarter of primary malignant bone tumours are osteosarcomas and metastasis to the lungs occurs early.
Chondrosarcoma	Arises from chondroblasts producing chondroid and collagen (not bone). It makes up 15% of malignant neoplasms arising from bone. Has a male predominance, usually over the age of 30, and most often occurring in proximal ends of long bones. Complete excision or amputation is usually curative with a 50% five-year survival. The tumour tends to become necrotic, showing bone destruction on X-ray.
Ewing's sarcoma	Arises in bone marrow in patients under the age of 30. Usually in long bones but occurs in flat bones in the older age group. A useful diagnostic characteristic is that it is not confined to the ends of the long bones. The site of the lesion usually exhibits tenderness.
Liposarcoma	A slow-growing tumour that invades widely, occurring in the fifth decade and affecting the buttock, thigh and shoulder regions.
Fibrosarcoma	A slow-growing soft-tissue tumour of muscle, ligament, tendon or periosteum, which metastasizes late and recurs locally.
Haemangiosarcoma	A rare soft-tissue tumour that usually regresses spontaneously.
Leiomyosarcoma	
Rhabdomyosarcoma	

What dictates how a sarcoma is typed?

It is typed by the greatest tissue volume that composes the tumour, or by the one that carries the worst prognosis. It is often of mixed type.

How is a sarcoma graded?

It is placed into one of four grades: well differentiated, moderately differentiated, poorly differentiated, or undifferentiated if no tissue can be identified (this grade usually carries the worst prognosis).

Scarring

What is a scar?

A scar is an area of fibrous tissue that is deposited during the healing process after a skin injury. It is a process of wound repair.

Name the main types of scarring

Wide scar –– This is commonly seen after limb or joint surgery; it is usually asymptomatic, flat and pale, occurring within weeks from surgery.

Hypertrophic scar –– This is commonly seen after a burn injury. The scar is usually raised and inflamed, and can be itchy and painful, but remains within the boundaries of the original injury. It generally regresses with time after the injury.

Keloid scar –– This commonly affects the shoulder region, sterna area and earlobes; it is seen most commonly in dark-skinned individuals. Keloid scars can be very itchy and painful, they can grow with time and do not regress spontaneously (compare with hypertrophic scars). It is raised and spreads beyond the margin of the wound, thus affecting normal surrounding skin. These scars invariably recur if excised and are difficult to manage.

Scar contracture –– This type of scaring commonly occurs when a wound crosses a joint, and is most common in burn injuries. It is of a hypertrophic type and can be very disabling. Contracture release should be carefully planned with an experienced plastic and reconstructive surgeon.

Tetanus

What is tetanus?

Tetanus is a disease of the central nervous system (CNS), causing painful uncontrolled muscle spasms.

It is caused by tetanospasmin ascending the motor nerve trunks and binding to the presynaptic inhibitory motor nerve endings. This prevents the release of the inhibitory neurotransmitters.

It results in muscle spasms and increased tone within the affected region, preceding any spread.

How does tetanospasmin get into the system?

- Spores of tetanus bacteria (*Clostridium tetani*) enter the body through an open wound or puncture wound, by injecting contaminated street drugs or through damage to the skin in a burn.
- It is found throughout the environment, usually in soil, dust, animal waste and metal rust.

What are the clinical signs of tetanus?

- Headache,
- Locked jaw – trismus,
- Muscle twitches, stiffness and spasms,
- Glottal spasm and dysphagia,
- Opisthotonus (extreme hyperextension),
- Hyperreflexia,
- Tetanic seizures,
- Approximately 30% of those who get infected die.

How soon after exposure do symptoms appear?

It varies from two days to months, but is usually less than two weeks. The earlier the symptoms appear, the more severe the infection.

How is it treated?

- Human antitetanus immunoglobulin (TIG): if the patient has not been immunized with the toxoid, it should be given as soon as possible after a tetanus-prone injury.
- This may cause anaphylaxis and only temporarily prevents the infection.

How is it prevented?

- Vaccination using denatured tetanus toxin to stimulate immunity, usually combined with diphtheria and pertussis vaccines (DTP).
- Five doses provide lifelong immunity.
- It does not prevent infection; it only prevents the toxin from activating the cascade of events.

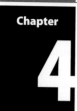

Chapter

Surgical skills and patient safety

Analgesia

What is the analgesic ladder?

- Non-opioid ± adjuvant (e.g. aspirin, paracetamol or non-steroid anti-inflammatory drugs (NSAIDs)),
- Mild opioid ± non-opioid ± adjuvant (e.g. codeine),
- Strong opioid ± non-opioid ± adjuvant (e.g. morphine, fentanyl).

How may analgesics be administered?

The common routes of administration are:

- Enteral: oral (including sublingual), rectal,
- Parenteral:
  - IV infusion, including patient-controlled analgesia (PCA),
  - Intermittent intramuscular injection or regional infiltration of local anaesthetic,
  - Intranasal, for opiates in the paediatric setting,
  - Intrathecal route: epidural analgesia using bupivacaine,
  - Inhalation, such as 70% nitrous oxide (a volatile anaesthetic),
  - Transcutaneous, such as fentanyl patches for chronic pain.

Give some examples of the opiates in common use. Which are the synthetic and non-synthetic agents?

The commonly used opiates are:

Non-synthetic	Morphine, codeine (10% of this is metabolized to morphine),
Semi-synthetic	Diamorphine, dihydrocodeine,
Synthetic	Pethidine, fentanyl.

Which receptor do opiate analgesics act on?

The majority of the effects of the opiates are carried out through the μ-receptor. They may also have some action through the other two types of opiate receptors, κ and δ.

What are the systemic effects of the opiates?

The effects of the opiates are:

Analgesia	They are good for moderate to severe pain of any cause and modality. They are less effective for neuropathic pain, such as phantom limb pain, or allodynia (pain from a non-painful stimulus).
Respiratory depression	Blunting of the ventilatory response to rising pCO_2 and suppression of the cough reflex; both of these encourage sputum retention, atelectasis and pneumonia in the critically ill.
Sedation	A reduction in the level of consciousness occurs with higher doses, so beware in patients with head injuries.
Nausea and vomiting	Following stimulation of the chemoreceptor trigger zones in the area postrema.
Reduced GI motility	This leads to constipation.
Euphoria	
Dependence and tolerance	There is a progressively reduced effect from the same dose of a drug.
Histamine release from mast cells	Producing pruritis and reduced systemic vascular resistance.

Why is morphine not advocated for use in abdominal pain of biliary origin?

Morphine increases the tone of the sphincter of Oddi (as well as other sphincteric muscles), while stimulating contraction of the gallbladder. Therefore, it can exacerbate biliary pain.

Which drug is given for opiate overdose? What is the mechanism of action?

Naloxone may be used to reverse the effects of opioids. This is a short-acting μ-receptor antagonist. Note that because of its short duration of action, the effects of the opioids may return after an initial reversal.

What are the therapeutic effects of paracetamol (acetaminophen)?

This is an analgesic and antipyretic with minimal anti-inflammatory properties.

By what mechanism does overdose cause liver injury?

The cause of liver injury lies with the metabolism of paracetamol. Normally it is conjugated in the liver, with the production of a small amount of the toxic metabolite: N-acetyl-benzoquinoneimine. Binding to hepatic glutathione receptors renders this metabolite harmless. With overdose, glutathione is depleted, leading to hepatocyte injury. Acetylcysteine, the drug used to treat overdose, is a glutathione precursor.

How do the non-steroidal anti-inflammatory drugs (NSAIDs) work?

These agents act to reduce prostaglandin formation by the inhibition of the enzyme cyclo-oxygenase, which acts on arachidonic acid. This leads to a modification of the inflammatory reaction and its effects on the stimulating nociception.

What are the systemic side effects of NSAIDs?

The systemic side effects of these agents include:

Gastrointestinal	Dyspepsia, gastritis and peptic ulceration. There is a direct stimulation of acid secretion by the gastric parietal cells, with reduced bicarbonate and mucus production.
Renal	NSAIDs may precipitate acute renal failure, especially in those with pre-existing renal suppression, dehydration or hypotension. Also leads to salt and water retention.
Coagulopathy	Inhibition of platelet thromboxane A_2 production leads to their reduced ability to aggregate and form the primary platelet plug. This is a permanent effect, and is reversed only when new platelets are formed.
Bronchospasm	The inhibition of cyclo-oxygenase leads to arachidonic acid being metabolized down the pathway of leucotriene formation, which induce bronchospasm.

How is renal injury precipitated?

There is inhibition of compensatory PGI2 and PGE2 formation that occurs during situations of reduced renal perfusion. These prostaglandins normally promote vasodilatation during such situations, offsetting the development of acute tubular necrosis.

What local anaesthetic techniques are available for pain relief?

The local anaesthetic techniques available are:

Local nerve blocks	Such as the three-in-one block of the lateral cutaneous, femoral and obturator nerves that can be used for fractured neck of femur. Also, an intercostal block following chest injury or thoracotomy.

Caudal block   Strictly speaking, a form of epidural anaesthesia; this is particularly useful for paediatric patients.

Epidural and spinal block   The former is more popular because of its longer duration of action and reduced systemic adverse effects. Spinal blocks are common in hip and knee surgery.

When is epidural analgesia commonly employed?

Epidural analgesia is commonly used in the postoperative setting, being especially useful in situations where pain may compromise respiratory function, e.g. thoracic or upper abdominal surgery.

Why is epidural analgesia's use limited in the critical care setting?

- The patient may be septic or have a local infection: both of which contraindicate the use of an epidural.
- Epidurals must not be inserted in the presence of a coagulopathy.
- The patient may not be able to consent owing to lack of consciousness.
- The patient may be hypovolaemic, leading to decompensated hypotension.

What are the potential systemic effects of this form of analgesia?

Some of the systemic effects of epidurals include:

- Hypotension, due to block of the sympathetic outflow causing peripheral vasodilatation,
- Reduced cardiac output due to a reduction in the venous return,
- Attenuation of the surgical stress response,
- Reduction of the functional residual capacity,
- Reduction of postoperative deep venous thrombosis for a number of reasons, including the concomitant use of IV fluids used to support the arterial pressure.

Diathermy

What different types of diathermy are available?

Monopolar (cutting, coagulation and blend) and bipolar (coagulation only). Both use alternating current (ac).

Give examples of uses of each

Monopolar diathermy is used in most general surgical procedures. Cutting diathermy may be used on dissection through soft tissues, whereas coagulation is often used on small vessels. Bipolar diathermy is used in extremity surgery to prevent high current densities over a small area of tissue (e.g. hands). It is also used in neurosurgical and plastic surgical procedures, where finer precision is required.

What is the difference between monopolar and bipolar diathermy?

Monopolar -- A high current density is produced at the tip of the diathermy probe, which then disseminates throughout the body as it is conducted to the diathermy plate (or indifferent electrode). To reduce the current density at the diathermy plate and prevent a heating effect, the diathermy plate must have a minimum surface area of 70 cm^2. Incorrect placement of the plate or contact with other conducting materials may result in burns. Power used is up to 400 W.

Bipolar -- The diathermy instrument consists of two electrodes (commonly combined as forceps) and current is conducted between the two electrodes; it only passes through the tissue that is being treated. It uses significantly lower power than monopolar diathermy and there is no need for a diathermy plate. Cutting is not possible with bipolar diathermy. Power used is up to 50 W.

Why does surgical diathermy not produce muscle stimulation?

No muscle stimulation is produced due to the high frequency of current in the diathermy circuit. The frequency of current used by diathermy units is 400 kHz to 10 MHz (mains frequency is 50 kHz). Muscle stimulation is produced at frequencies of <50 kHz and at this frequency even small currents (5–10 mA) may cause muscle stimulation. The use of higher frequencies therefore also allows much higher currents to be safely conducted through tissues.

What is the difference between the cutting and coagulation settings? What other settings may be used?

Cutting -- A continuous current output allows arcing of the current between the tip of the electrode and the tissue. This creates a temperature of approximately 1000 °C in the local tissue, resulting in vaporization of cell water and tissue disruption. There is little coagulation when this setting is used.

Coagulation -- A pulsed current output is generated, resulting in local heat production with tissue desiccation and sealing of blood vessels. There is minimal tissue disruption.

Other available settings include fulguration (spray coagulation) and blend. Fulguration uses a high voltage to coagulate over a wider area. Blend produces a continuous output with pulses that allows simultaneous coagulation and cutting.

What are the risks associated with diathermy?

1. Incorrect plate position may result in burns, owing to poor heat dissipation. The plate must be positioned over areas with good blood supply and away from bony prominences, scar tissue and metal implants.

2. Large bowel gas and alcoholic skin preparations that are not sufficiently allowed to dry may result in explosion.

3. There is potential for diathermy smoke to contain carcinogens. Direct inhalation should be avoided.

4. Use of monopolar diathermy on appendages may result in setting up high current density locally (without the ability to dissipate current) causing tissue damage distant from the site of the electrode.

5. The use of diathermy adjacent to metal implants or other metal objects may allow current to be induced in a metal object without direct contact between it and the diathermy electrode. This could result in heating around the metal object and tissue damage.

6 Capacitance coupling: the diathermy electrode comprises a metal active wire surrounded by an insulating layer. In laparoscopic surgery, this is then contained within a metal cannula, which passes through a port (either metal or plastic) into the abdominal cavity. In this set-up, ac current may be conducted from the active wire to the surrounding metal cannula without direct contact, as the insulating layer acts as the capacitor. The stray current is then dissipated through the patient's body to the diathermy plate, provided that the cannula is housed within a metal port. The current density is usually low and little or no heating effect occurs around the port site. If however, a metal cannula is used with a non-conducting port there will be no discharge current from the cannula before its entry into the abdominal cavity. This may result in damage to structures (e.g. the bowel) that are in contact with the cannula but out of view.

7. Direct coupling: if the electrode is in contact with another metal object, this will result in conduction of current through this object and may cause heating and damage to adjacent tissues.

What contraindications do you know to the use of diathermy?

Pacemakers or implantable cardioverter defibrillators (ICDs). Diathermy should be avoided where possible, and if needed a bipolar circuit should be used. Monopolar diathermy may cause:

1. Induced current down the pacemaker wires, resulting in myocardial burns.

2. Induced currents in the logic circuits of the pacemaker, resulting in potential change to pacing rate or inhibition of output. An ICD may be inappropriately stimulated, owing to misinterpretation of an interference signal as myocardial activity. Both these instances may result in fatal arrhythmias.

Knee aspiration

Why is a knee aspiration performed?

To aid diagnosis, relieve discomfort or drain infected fluid, and for intra-articular drug delivery.

What are the indications of knee aspiration?

- Septic joint (isolate an organism via microscopy and culture),
- Crystal-induced arthropathy (includes gout and pseudogout),
- Haemarthrosis (relative),
- Unexplained monoarthrosis or effusion,
- Symptomatic relief from large tense effusion.

What are the key aspects in performing a knee aspiration?

After a physical examination and establishing the presence of an effusion, the patient is placed supine and the knee either extended or flexed at 90°. The supra-lateral aspect of the knee joint (1 cm superior and lateral to the supra-lateral aspect of the patella) provides the best access to the synovium. This area should be marked with a pen. After the skin has been prepared and draped appropriately, using an aseptic technique, infiltrate the skin producing a 'bleb' of local anaesthetic, then infiltrate the tissues more deeply down to the level of the synovial membrane of the suprapatellar pouch (but not through the synovium). The aspiration needle (usu-ally a sterile 21-gauge needle or a cannula if the effusion is large to ease evacuation) is inserted at 45° distally and 45° towards and underneath the patella. During the procedure, the free hand could compress the opposite side to aid the aspiration. Once complete, the needle-puncture site should be cleaned and dressed.

The same technique is used for intra-articular joint injection with local anaesthetic and steroid.

What does a haemarthrosis within the knee joint indicate?

It indicates a significant injury that could include a fracture that communi-cates with the joint, or a significant ligament injury, such as an anterior cruciate ligament rupture (vascular structure).

Why should you not inject local anaesthetic into the joint prior to aspiration of a potentially septic knee?

Many local anaesthetics (e.g., lignocaine) have bactericidal properties, which would interfere with culture accuracy.

Nerve injuries

What are the different layers within peripheral nerves? *(From out to in)*

- External epineurium,
- Internal epineurium,
- Fascicular groups (consisting of perineurium),
- Fascicles (consisting of endoneurium),
- Nerve fibres (consisting of Schwann's cells making up the myelin sheath),
- Axon.

What are the common causes of nerve injury?

Direct trauma –– Laceration, gunshot injuries, penetrating injuries, burns, blunt trauma, iatrogenic (e.g., during operative fixation of fractures, traction or direct laceration).

Indirect trauma –– Secondary to fracture fragments, dislocations, compartment syndrome, iatrogenic (e.g., prolonged tourniquet use).

What physiological changes occurs following nerve injury?

Wallerian degeneration –– The nerve will begin to degrade in an anterograde fashion. The axon and surrounding myelin break down during this process. The round mast cells can be seen, as can the phagocytic macrophages that interact with Schwann's cells to remove the injured tissue debris. As the degradation of the distal nerve segment continues, connection with the target muscle is lost, leading to muscle atrophy and fibrosis. Once the degenerative events are complete, all that remains is a column of collapsed Schwann's cells (bands of Büngner). Axon sprouts, each with a finger-like growth cone, advance using the Schwann's cells as guides. After reinnervation, the newly connected axon matures and the pre-injury cytoarchitecture and function are restored.

What are the types of nerve injury?

Figure 4.1 illustrates the classification system for injuries of the peripheral nervous system.

Neuropraxia –– This is the least severe nerve injury; it heals with full recovery of function (usually within six to eight weeks). Conduction within the nerve proximal and distal to the injury remains intact, as does the continuity of the structures. There is no Wallerian degeneration in this type of injury, but there is focal demyelination. *Good prognosis.*

Axonotmesis –– Is a more severe injury, with damage to the myelin sheath and disruption to the axon, but the peri- and epineurium remain intact. Wallerian degeneration occurs distal to the injury, and recovery is good but may require many months. *Fair prognosis.*

Neurotmesis –– This is the most severe nerve injury. There is complete disruption to the axons, endo-, peri- and epineurium. Wallerian degeneration occurs and axonal regeneration does not take place. Recovery requires surgical repair and apposition of the nerve. Prognosis is variable from complete to no recovery. *Poor prognosis.*

What is the growth rate of injured peripheral nerves?

1 mm/day.

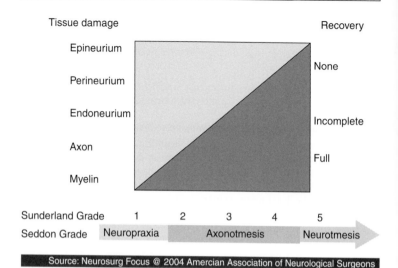

Figure 4.1 Classification of injuries of the peripheral nervous system.

What factors influence the degree of recovery in significant nerve injury?

- Age of patient,
- Type of injury,
- Degree of injury,
- Level of injury (proximity to cell body has worse prognosis, owing to cell death),
- Associated injuries and the condition of the injured nerve.

What is the cause of nerve injuries secondary to patient positioning in theatre?

This is caused by local nerve ischaemia following direct pressure or compression or traction or stretching. This is more commonly seen in prolonged surgery.

What are the common nerve injuries secondary to patient positioning in theatre for a procedure under general anaesthesia?

Brachial plexus –– Injury is caused by excessive stretching usually by arm abduction (>90°), external rotation and posterior shoulder displacement, but can also occur in excessive extension and lateral flexion of the head. Care needs to be taken during prone positioning of patients in spinal procedures.

Ulnar nerve –– As the nerve is very superficial along the posterior aspect of the medial epicondyle of the humerus, it is vulnerable to compression against the operating table, especially if the arm is extended and pronated.

Radial nerve -- Lesion usually results secondary to compression of the nerve between the edge of the operating table or arm board and humerus, as well as when the patient is in the lateral position.

Sciatic nerve -- Injury is uncommon but the risk is greatest in thin patients undergoing long operations in a lateral position over a hard unpadded table. The sciatic nerve is also vulnerable to stretching in the lithotomy position.

Common peroneal nerve -- The risk is similar to the sciatic nerve but much more common. Lithotomy position is the most common mechanism of injury by compression of the nerve around the fibula head.

Of the nerve injuries listed, which are the most commonly seen?

Upper limb -- Ulnar nerve at the elbow.

Lower limb -- Common peroneal nerve at the knee.

What are the complications of nerve injury?

A patient can develop clinical features of anaesthesia, paraesthesia, hyperaesthesia (including chronic regional pain syndrome), and pain around the areas supplied by the nerve. Paresis and paralysis can occur. This can also lead to muscle wasting, joint stiffness and demineralization of bone. Laceration of nerve can lead to the development of neuromas.

Principles of fracture management

What is the main aim of fracture management?

Reduce the fracture; *immobilize* the fracture in a satisfactory position; followed by *rehabilitation*.

What are the options in fracture reduction?

Closed reduction -- This is the non-operative route in fracture reduction. This can be done with analgesia and local anaesthetics (such as using a haematoma block: local anaesthesia in the fracture site) followed by traction and counter-traction on the limb in question. This manipulation can also be done under general anaesthetic in a theatre setting if indicated.

Open reduction -- If closed reduction fails or is inappropriate, open reduction may be used. This entails the operative route followed by fixation to hold the fracture.

What are the known methods of immobilization?

Non-operative

Splints	Neighbour strapping of fingers and toes; various forms of splint are available.

| Cast | Using either plaster of Paris or synthetic fibreglass material (lightweight). They can be full casts or back-slabs (half casts used especially in the acute phase of the injury to allow for soft tissue swelling). |
| Traction | This can be in the form of skin traction or skeletal traction (using a pin, which can be inserted under local or general anaesthetic) with weights to maintain the force exerted on the limb. |

Operative: internal fixation

| Intramedullary | Nail devices that are inserted into the medulla of the bone. |
| Extramedullary | Kirschner wires (K-wires) or plate and screws, which involve at least one cortex of the bone. |

Operative: external fixation

Various types of frames, usually held with Schanz screws: uniplanar, biplanar, delta (and other combinations), circular (such as an Ilizarov frame), hybrid frames (include tensioned wires, commonly used for distal tibial fractures).

Describe the importance of mobilization during rehabilitation

During the period of immobilization, continuous movement of all other joints is essential to prevent stiffness and especially in the lower limbs, to prevent deep vein thrombosis secondary to stasis.

Physiotherapy and occupational therapy play an integral role in this process of rehabilitation. Once the cast is removed, functional braces, which provide limb support with the ability of early light movement within the affected joint, are often seen as an option, to prevent complications of stiffness and immobility.

Skin preparation and asepsis

What different types of skin preparation solutions are you aware of?

The solutions most commonly used are:

10% Povidone-iodine –– Bactericidal as well as bacteriostatic, with little irritation to skin or mucosa. It can be used as a skin preparation solution and in areas where the skin is breached.

Chlorhexidine 0.5% in 70% alcohol –– Bactericidal and bacteriostatic, although reduced bactericidal effect with some gram-negative bacteria. Care should be taken to allow alcohol preparation solutions to dry before the use of electrocautery, as there is a risk that vapour may ignite.

What are the most commonly used surgical scrub solutions?

Povidone iodine 7.5% (Betadine) and Chlorhexidine gluconate 4%.

What is the difference between sterilization and disinfection?

Sterilization is defined as a process by which all microorganisms (bacteria, fungi and viruses) are destroyed. Disinfection is a process in which infective microorganisms are removed (bacteria, fungi and viruses).

What are the different methods of sterilization?

Steam (via autoclave) -- Autoclaves produce moist heat, combining temperature and pressure. Requirements to achieve sterilization are 134 °C for 3 min at 2 kPa or 121 °C for 15 min at 1 kPa. Autoclaving does not necessarily eliminate prions (usually treated with sodium hydroxide for two hours plus autoclaving for one hour at 160 °C).

Dry heat -- Requires much longer duration than moist heat; used for moisture-sensitive objects. Requirements for sterilization are at least 2 hours at 160 °C or 6–12 minutes at 190 °C.

Ethylene oxide -- Used in heat sensitive objects: it kills all known bacteria, spores, fungi and viruses. The disadvantages are that it requires a longer period of sterilization, requires poststerilization aeration to remove toxic residues and is highly flammable.

Peracetic acid (0.2%) -- Used in sterilization of endoscopes.

Radiation -- Gamma radiation is used for industrial sterilization of instruments and other equipment (cannulae, syringes, giving sets, etc.). Not used on a small scale, owing to the requirements for housing and safe use of gamma radioisotopes.

What systems are in place in the operating theatre to reduce the risk of infection?

Laminar flow operating rooms -- Air cycles with a minimum of 300 changes per hour. Used in orthopaedic theatres to reduce the risk of implant infection (some studies have shown a fourfold reduction).

Positive pressure ventilation -- Approximately 20 changes per hour. Higher pressure in the clean areas and lower pressure in the dirty areas results in flow of air from clean to dirty areas. This reduces the bacterial count in clean areas.

Suture materials and needles

What different types of suture do you know of?

Suture materials may be categorized as (1) natural, synthetic and metallic, (2) absorbable or non-absorbable, or (3) monofilament or multifilament.

Give examples of natural, synthetic and metallic sutures and their uses

Natural sutures

Catgut   Not used as has been banned in Europe and Japan, owing to concerns about transmission of prion disease.

Silk   General soft tissue closure and ligation. Avoid in vascular anastamoses and skin closure, owing to formation of stitch sinuses and abscesses.

Synthetic sutures

Vicryl/Vicryl Rapide (polyglactin)	Soft tissue and fascial closure. Also used in tendon repair. Vicryl Rapide commonly used in paediatric skin closure.
PDS (polydioxanone)	Mass closure of midline laparotomy incision.
Proline (polypropylene)	Closure of facial wounds and vascular anastamoses.
Ethilon (nylon, polyamide)	In ligation or in general soft tissue approximation, and skin closure in trauma.

Metallic sutures

Steel   Closure of the sternum after median sternotomy.

How would you classify sutures according to absorbability?

Absorbable   Vicryl/Vicryl Rapide, PDS, catgut.

Non-absorbable   Prolene, nylon, silk, steel.

Over what period do the absorbable sutures degenerate?

Vicryl -- Complete absorption at 56–70 days. Retains 40% of its tensile strength at 4 weeks.

Vicryl Rapide -- Complete absorption at 42 days. Retains 0% of its tensile strength at 10–14 days.

PDS -- Completely hydrolysed at 182–238 days. Retains 35–60% of its tensile strength at 6 weeks (depending on size of suture).

Chromic catgut -- Full tensile strength remains for 7–10 days and is fully hydrolysed at 90 days. Pure catgut is absorbed more quickly and causes an intense tissue reaction.

Give examples of monofilament and multifilament sutures

Monofilament -- PDS, prolene, nylon

Multifilament -- Vicryl or Vicryl Rapide, silk, catgut.

What are the advantages and disadvantages of monofilament sutures?

Advantages -- Less tissue reaction; glides easily; infection is less likely to settle in between the filaments, as may occur with braided sutures; less platelet activation (ideal for vascular anastamoses).

Disadvantages -- Monofilament sutures often have memory and can be difficult to handle and tie; therefore, more throws are required to form a secure knot.

Summarize the sizing of suture materials

Suture sizes are defined by the United States Pharmacopeia (USP) scale. This scale uses zero as the baseline. As the suture diameter decreases below the baseline, zeros are added, e.g. 0000 or 4-0). As the suture diameter increases above the baseline, a number is given to denote the size (e.g. number 4). The smallest available suture is 11-0 (0.01 mm diameter) and is used in microsurgery and ophthalmology. The largest is a braided number 5 suture (0.7 mm diameter), which is often used in orthopaedic surgery.

What types of needles are available? Give examples

Needles may be straight, curved or J-shaped. These may then be further categorized according to the body and the point of the needle. The body may be cutting, reverse-cutting or round-bodied. The point may be cutting, blunt or tapered. A forward-cutting needle has the sharp edge on the inside of the curve and a reverse-cutting needle has the cutting edge on the outside (preventing inside cut-out). Round-bodied, blunt needles are used in tissues that may be easily penetrated and damaged (e.g. in mass closure of abdominal midline laparotomy incisions, to prevent damage to the underlying bowel).

Tourniquet

What gases must never be used in pneumatic tourniquets?

Oxygen and nitrous oxide. Air is the gas that is normally used.

How much overlap must there be when applying the cuff, and what are the consequences of too much overlap?

7.5–15 cm. Too much overlap leads to increased pressure and rolling or wrinkling of tissue beneath, which can increase the risk of tourniquet complications.

Why is a large cuff width preferred and where should it be positioned?

A larger cuff width would be more effective in occluding blood flow at lower pressure, and it should be positioned at the point of greatest diameter. Caution should be taken in overweight or obese patients owing to the conical shape of the limb, and therefore contoured cuffs should be used, as they are able to occlude arterial flow at lower pressures more effectively.

What is the definition of limb occlusion pressure (LOP) and how is it calculated?

This is the minimum pressure required, at a specific time in a specific tourniquet cuff applied to a specific patient's limb at a specific location, to stop the flow of arterial blood into the limb distal to the cuff.

It can be calculated by two ways:

1. Cuff pressure can be increased slowly from zero while monitoring the pulse in an artery distal to the cuff until the distal pulse disappears; the lowest cuff pressure at which the pulse disappears can be defined as the ascending LOP.

2. Cuff pressure can be decreased slowly (1 mmHg/s) from a high occlusive level while monitoring an artery distal to the cuff until a distal pulse resumes; the highest pressure at which pulsatile flow first resumes can be defined as the descending LOP.

The mean of the ascending and descending LOP can be used as an estimate of the true LOP.

How is tourniquet pressure set based on LOP in adults in upper and lower limbs?

Upper limb tourniquet pressure = LOP + 50 mmHg,

Lower limb tourniquet pressure = LOP + 75 mmHg.

What is an alternative method of setting the tourniquet pressure in adults in upper and lower limbs?

Upper limb 50–75 mmHg above the patient's systolic BP,

Lower limb 100–150 mmHg above the patient's systolic BP.

List four adverse reactions to tourniquet over-pressurization

- Pain at the cuff site,
- Muscle weakness,
- Compression injuries to blood vessels, nerves, muscle, or skin,
- Extremity paralysis.

List five adverse reactions to tourniquet under-pressurization

- Blood in the surgical field,
- Passive congestion of the limb,
- Deep vein thrombosis,

- Shock,
- Haemorrhagic infiltration of a nerve.

What is the recommended maximum inflation time for the upper and lower limbs?

Upper limb   1 h,
Lower limb   1.5–2 h.

What adverse reactions could result if inflation time is prolonged?

- Excessive hyperaemia,
- Muscle weakness,
- Ischaemic injury,
- Extremity paralysis.

What is the minimum reperfusion time before the tourniquet can be re-inflated?

If you were to re-inflate a tourniquet after a prolonged period of usage, reperfusion of the limb should be for 10 minutes.

What are two relative contraindications to pneumatic tourniquet use?

Peripheral vascular disease and open fractures.

What minimum information must be documented in the notes regarding pneumatic tourniquets?

- Pressure inflated to,
- Limb used on,
- Duration of inflation.

When must limb exsanguination not be used before inflating the tourniquet cuff?

- Skin fragility,
- Infection,
- Thrombi,
- Malignant tumours.

What are three methods of exsanguinating a limb?

- Rhys Davies,
- Esmarch's bandage,
- Elevation.

Why is it important to prevent fluids from leaking beneath the cuff and why must it be inflated rapidly?

Fluid leaking under the cuff can result in chemical burn. Inflating the cuff rapidly prevents venous pooling in the segment distal to cuff, which could lead to thrombus formation.

What biochemical abnormalities may result after prolonged tourniquet times (>2 h)?

- Increased K^+,
- Increased lactate,
- Transient acidosis.

What is post-tourniquet syndrome? How long does the tourniquet need to be on for this to occur?

After tourniquet times of 2–4 hours, stiffness, pallor, weakness without paralysis and subjective numbness of the extremity can occur.

What precaution must be taken if local anaesthetic is administered at a point distal to the cuff?

Deflate slowly to prevent sudden bolus of local anaesthetic release into blood stream.

What two tissues are at greatest risk of damage as a result of tourniquet use?

- Muscle,
- Nerves.

Basic science

Anatomy

5

Anatomical snuffbox

What is the anatomical snuffbox?

The anatomical snuffbox (Figure 5.1) is a triangular deepening on the dorsal aspect of the wrist on the radial side. The name originates from the use of this surface for placing and sniffing 'snuff' or powdered tobacco in the past.

What are the boundaries of the anatomical snuffbox?

Radial Parallel tendons of extensor pollicis brevis and abductor pollicis longus,

Ulnar Tendon of extensor pollicis longus,

Floor Tip of radial styloid, scaphoid (majority) and trapezium, and the base of the thumb metacarpal (proximal to distal).

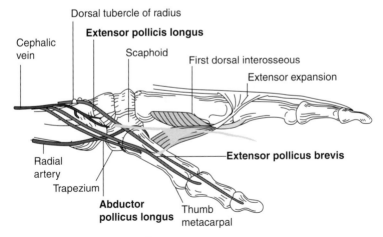

Dorsal tubercle of radius
Extensor pollicis longus
Cephalic vein
Scaphoid
First dorsal interosseous
Extensor expansion
Radial artery
Extensor pollicus brevis
Trapezium
Abductor pollicus longus
Thumb metacarpal

Figure 5.1 The anatomical snuffbox.

What neurovascular structures lie within this area?

- Radial artery (deep),
- Dorsal cutaneous branch of the radial nerve,
- Cephalic vein (superficial).

What does tenderness in the anatomical snuffbox classically signify?

Fracture of the scaphoid. This is most commonly caused from a fall onto the outstretched hand in a young adult.

What is particular about the blood supply of the scaphoid and what is its significance?

The proximal segment of the scaphoid lacks any independent blood supply. The blood supply of the scaphoid comes from the radial artery. It is characteristic in the fact that it supplies the bone from distal to proximal. Therefore, a fracture through the waist of the scaphoid may result in avascular necrosis (AVN) of the proximal pole. The more proximal the fracture position, the higher the risk of AVN.

What other bones have a risk of developing AVN?

The femoral head and the talus.

Antecubital fossa and elbow joint

Where is the cubital fossa situated and what are its boundaries?

The cubital fossa (Figure 5.2) is a triangular area found on the anterior aspect of the elbow,[1] with its base (superior border) forming a line between the medial and lateral epicondyles.

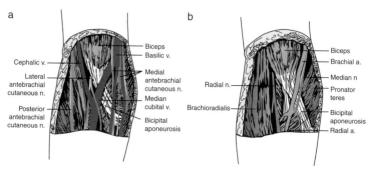

Figure 5.2 The cubital fossa. (a) The superficial nerves and veins. (b) The contents of the cubital fossa.

---

[1] www.joint-pain-expert.net/elbow-anatomy.html.

Medial (ulnar) border	Lateral aspect of pronator teres (a muscle that pronates and flexes the forearm), innervated by the median nerve.
Lateral (radial) border	Medial aspect of brachioradialis muscle (another forearm flexor, commonly known as the 'beer drinkers' muscle'), innervated by the radial nerve.
Apex	The tip of the triangle is directed distally and is formed by the meeting point of the medial and lateral boundaries.
Floor (deep)	Brachialis muscle and supinator.
Roof (superficial)	Deep fascia reinforced by the bicipital aponeurosis, superficial fascia (containing the median cubital vein and the medial and lateral cutaneous nerves of the forearm) and skin.

What are the contents of the cubital fossa?

Lateral to medial present in the fossa in a vertical configuration:

Radial nerve	Found between the brachioradialis and brachialis – this nerve is not always considered to be part of the cubital fossa.
Biceps brachii tendon	Can be palpated clinically.
Brachial artery	Distal aspect of the artery and the bifurcation (at the apex of the triangle) into the radial and ulnar arteries.
Median nerve	

If excluding the radial nerve, the mnemonic TAN ('tendon artery nerve') can be applied from lateral to medial.

The ulnar nerve is in the vicinity of the cubital fossa but not considered to be within the fossa. It is found medial to the median nerve.

The median cubital, cephalic and basilic veins, and the medial and lateral cutaneous nerve are considered to be superficial to the cubital fossa. However, they are important structures to bear in mind in any laceration or fracture that involves the region around the cubital fossa.

What clinical aspects are useful with the anatomical knowledge of the cubital fossa?

- Palpation of the brachial pulse, in addition to manual blood pressure measurements with the stethoscope places over the brachial artery,
- Peripheral venous cannulation and phlebotomy,

- Assessment of neurovascular injuries in any fracture involving this region, especially supracondylar fractures in children with increased threat to these structures (most common is the median nerve's anterior interosseous branch, followed by the ulnar and radial).

What type of joint is the elbow joint?

It is a synovial hinge joint. It consists of the distal humerus articulating with both the proximal radius and ulna. Stability of the joint is reinforced by the concavity of the olecranon and its articulation with the trochlea. Various ligaments around the elbow joint also aid stability. Given the nature of the hinge joint, the movements that are produced around the elbow are of flexion and extension. Pronation and supination of the forearm and movements that are produced from the radioulnar joints despite the articulation of the radial head with the capitellum.

Arterial supply of the lower limb

What are the main branches of the arterial blood supply to the lower limb?

See Figure 5.3.

- The *external iliac artery* (bifurcation of the *common iliac artery*) becomes the femoral artery at the point beyond the inguinal ligament.
- The *femoral artery* anatomically begins at the mid-inguinal point (midway between the anterior superior iliac spine (ASIS) and the symphysis pubis).
- The femoral artery then bifurcates into the superficial femoral artery and the profunda femoris. This division occurs just below the femoral sheath.
- The *superficial femoral artery* continues into the adductor canal and forms the popliteal artery in the adductor hiatus as it goes into the popliteal fossa.
- The *profunda femoris* is the main blood supply of the thigh and runs deep in the thigh. It branches into the medial and lateral circumflex femoral arteries to supply the proximal thigh and the hip joint, as well as three or four perforating arteries.
- After the formation of the *popliteal artery* at the adductor hiatus, it runs deep in the popliteal fossa and along the medial aspect of the femur, almost in contact with bone. It lies at the posterior capsule of the knee as it travels distally in the fossa.
- The popliteal artery branches into two *genicular arteries* on the lateral aspect of the knee and three medially (the middle genicular artery supplies the cruciate ligaments).
- The popliteal artery divides into the *anterior and posterior tibial arteries*. The anterior tibial artery continues as the *dorsalis pedis* artery after it

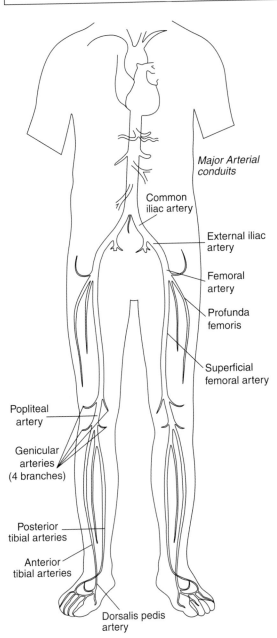

Figure 5.3
Arterial supply of
the lower limb.

Major Arterial conduits

Common iliac artery

External iliac artery

Femoral artery

Profunda femoris

Superficial femoral artery

Popliteal artery

Genicular arteries (4 branches)

Posterior tibial arteries

Anterior tibial arteries

Dorsalis pedis artery

crosses the ankle anteriorly, beneath the extensor retinaculum and midway between both malleoli. It finally forms the dorsal arch artery of the foot. The posterior tibial artery is the main blood supply to the foot and runs posterior to the medial malleolus. It finally branches into the medial and lateral plantar arteries.

Carpal tunnel

Where is the carpal tunnel situated and what are its attachments?

The carpal tunnel (Figure 5.4) is situated in the upper limb. It is a space on the volar surface of the wrist between the concavity of the carpus and the overlying flexor retinaculum. The flexor retinaculum (carpal ligament) is a strong fibrous band the size of a postage stamp. The proximal edge of the flexor retinaculum underlies the distal wrist crease.

Attachments of the flexor retinaculum:

Radial aspect	Proximally the scaphoid tubercle and distally the ridge of trapezium.
Ulnar aspect	Proximally the pisiform (sesamoid bone within flexor carpi ulnaris) and distally the hook of hamate.

What are the contents of the carpal tunnel?

Median nerve	Most superficial; just beneath the retinaculum radial to midpoint,
Flexor pollicis longus (FPL)	Has its own synovial sheath; runs radial to finger flexors,

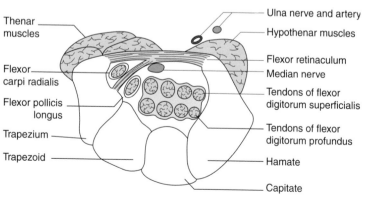

Figure 5.4 A diagrammatic cross-section through the carpal tunnel.

Flexor carpi radialis (FCR)	Within its own fascial compartment and radial to finger flexors,
Flexor digitorum superficialis (FDS)	Running in two pairs,
Flexor digitorum profundus (FDP)	Running more dorsal to flexor digitorum superficialis, in a row of four.

Compartments of the lower limb

How many compartments are there in the lower limb?

Four: anterior, lateral, superficial posterior and deep posterior (see Figure 5.5).

What are the contents of the anterior compartment of the lower leg?

The anterior compartment lies between the deep fascia of the anterior aspect of the lower leg and the interosseous membrane between the tibia and fibula. Its contents include:

- Tibialis anterior,
- Extensor hallucis longus,
- Extensor digitorum longus,
- Peroneus tertius,
- Anterior tibial artery,
- Deep peroneal nerve.

What are the contents of the lateral compartment of the lower leg?

- Peroneus longus,
- Peroneus brevis,
- Branches of the peroneal artery,
- Superficial peroneal nerve.

What are the contents of the posterior compartment of the lower leg?

Superficial
- Gastrocnemius,
- Soleus,
- Plantaris,
- Underlying deep transverse fascia separating superficial from deep.

Deep
- Tibialis posterior,
- Flexor digitorum longus,
- Flexor hallucis longus,

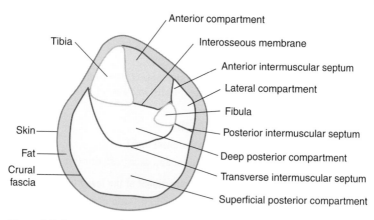

Figure 5.5 Cross-section through the middle third of the leg.

- Popliteus,
- Posterior tibial artery,
- Peroneal artery,
- Tibial nerve,
- Sural nerve.

Dermatomes and myotomes of the upper and lower limb

What are dermatomes?

Dermatomes (Figure 5.6) are areas of skin that are supplied by a single posterior spinal nerve root. They can be identified in examinations of the limbs.

Dermatomes of the upper limb

    C4   Shoulder tip,

    C5   Outer part of the upper arm,

    C6   Lateral aspect of the forearm and the thumb,

    C7   Middle finger,

    C8   Little finger,

    T1   Medial aspect of the upper arm.

Other useful dermatomes on the trunk

    T4   Nipples,

    T7   Xiphisternum,

    T10 Level of umbilicus.

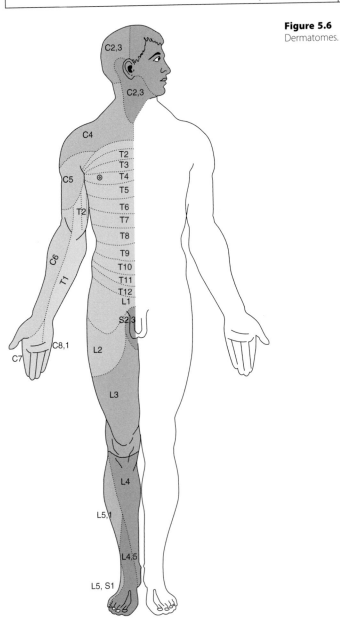

Figure 5.6
Dermatomes.

Dermatomes of the lower limb

L1 Around inguinal region and anterior perineum,

L3 Front of knee,

L4 Over tibia/medial leg,

L5 Over fibula/lateral leg,

L5 Medial side of foot,

S1 Lateral side of foot.

One stands on S1, sits on S3 (around the anus) and S2 is a narrow strip up the middle of the calf and hamstrings.

Note that there are extensive overlaps between dermatomes and therefore various references will have slight variations of the exact mapping of the dermatomes. These maps are a guide to ease examination and aid in diagnosis.

Femoral triangle

What are the boundaries of the femoral triangle?

See Figure 5.7.

Superiorly Inguinal ligament,

Medially Medial border of adductor longus muscle,

Laterally Medial border of sartorius muscle,

Floor Iliacus, tendon of pectineus, psoas and adductor longus,

Roof Superficial fascia and fascia lata.

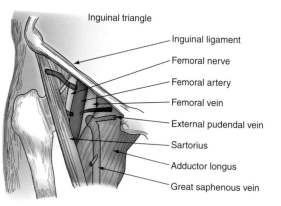

Inguinal triangle

— Inguinal ligament

— Femoral nerve

— Femoral artery

— Femoral vein

— External pudendal vein

— Sartorius

— Adductor longus

— Great saphenous vein

Figure 5.7
Femoral triangle.

What are the contents of the femoral triangle?

From lateral to medial:

- Femoral nerve,
- Femoral artery,
- Femoral vein,
- Femoral canal (containing extra-peritoneal fat and Cloquet's lymph node), and
- Deep inguinal lymph nodes within the femoral triangle.

What operative procedures occur in and around the femoral triangle?

Femoral embolectomy for acute limb ischaemia, and femoral hernia repairs.

Hip and femur

See Figure 5.8.

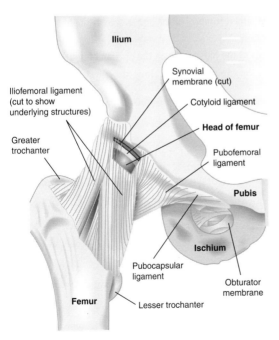

Figure 5.8 Hip and femur.

Ilium

Synovial membrane (cut)

Iliofemoral ligament (cut to show underlying structures)

Cotyloid ligament

Head of femur

Greater trochanter

Pubofemoral ligament

Pubis

Ischium

Pubocapsular ligament

Obturator membrane

Femur

Lesser trochanter

What kind of joint is the acetabulofemoral joint?

The hip joint is a synovial ball-and-socket joint lined by hyaline cartilage, involving the acetabulum and femur.

What are the factors that contribute to the intrinsic stability of the hip?

All three factors of the bony, ligamentous and muscular components affect and contribute to the stability of the hip. Note that while performing a total hip replacement (THR) some of these factors are compromised; therefore, there is a risk of dislocation.

Osseous –– The ball and socket, which is further deepened by the labrum, are the primary stabilizing factors.

Ligamentous –– Including the capsule, there are three main ligaments – iliofemoral, pubofemoral and ischiofemoral. The iliofemoral (strongest ligament) is shaped like an inverted Y, originating from above the anterior superior iliac spine (ASIS) with the limbs of the Y attaching around the intertrochanteric line. The pubofemoral ligament is found at the inferior joint capsule between the iliopubic eminence and the obturator crest. The ischiofemoral ligament (weakest ligament) winds around the joint and attaches into the capsule.

Muscular –– The short lateral rotators of the hip, as well as the hip abductors (gluteus medius and minimus).

What are the attachments of the hip capsule on the proximal femur?

On the anterior aspect, the capsule attaches along the intertrochanteric line. Posteriorly, it attaches more proximally halfway along the femoral neck. Superiorly, it is attached circumferentially around the labrum and the transverse ligament.

What is the shape of the acetabulum?

The acetabulum is a concave surface of the pelvis with a horseshoe-shaped articular surface. The acetabular labrum is attached to the rim of the acetabulum to deepen the socket (it is triangular in cross-section). The transverse acetabular ligament is found between the two limbs of the horseshoe.

What three bones form the acetabulum?

- Ischium,
- Ilium,
- Pubis.

If given a femur how do you orientate it to the correct side?

- Femoral condyles face posteriorly,
- Linea aspera is posterior,

- Lesser trochanter is medial and posterior,
- Femoral neck and head angled supero-medially, and from posterior to anterior.

Where does the iliopsoas muscle attach on the femur and what is its action?

The iliopsoas (iliacus and psoas major muscles) inserts to the lesser trochanter. Its action is to flex the hip.

What does tenderness at the greater trochanter commonly indicate without the presence of an acute injury?

Trochanteric bursitis.

What muscles attach to the linea aspera at the posterior aspect of the femur?

The linea aspera is extended by three ridges superiorly and two ridges posteriorly.

Superior third
- Pectineus,
- Iliacus,
- Adductor longus,
- Adductor brevis.

Middle third
- Gluteus maximus,
- Short head of biceps femoris.

Inferior third
- Adductor magnus,
- Vastus lateralis and medialis.

Knee joint

What type of bone is the patella?

The patella is a sesamoid bone. It is the largest sesamoid bone in the body, lying within the tendon of the quadriceps, which attaches at the tibial tubercle.

What shape is the patella?

The patella is circular-triangular, with its apex facing distally. It articulates with the distal femur (the articular surface of the knee joint). The cartilaginous posterior surface is divided by a vertical ridge into a larger lateral portion for articulation with the lateral condyle of the femur and a smaller medial portion for articulation with the medial condyle of femur.

What is the common age of patella subluxation or dislocation?

It can occur in childhood but is more common in adolescence and early adulthood (16–20). It is also seen more commonly in young female athletes.

In what direction does the patella usually dislocate?

Laterally.

What are the predisposing factors for patella subluxation or dislocation?

Age	16–20,
Sex	Female,
Athletic population	Particularly in twisting rotational motions of the knee, or direct trauma to the knee,
Family history	
Anatomic factors	Insufficient oblique insertion of vastus medialis (VMO) muscle, laxity or injury to the medial patellofemoral ligament (MPFL), misalignment of the patella, patella alta or dysplastic patella shallow trochlear groove and decreased prominence of the lateral femoral condyle.

Describe the attachments of the capsule of the knee

Anteriorly, the synovial membrane is attached to the femur proximal to the articular surface, while distally on the tibia the attachment is near the articular cartilage. Posteriorly, the femoral attachments lie at the cartilaginous margin of the medial and lateral femoral condyles, with the tibial attachments similarly at the cartilage margin.

What are the attachments of the cruciate ligaments of the knee?

The anterior and posterior cruciate ligaments (ACL and PCL) are named after their points of attachment on the tibial plateau.

Anterior cruciate ligament –– This originates from the medial wall (posterior part) of the lateral femoral condyle and attaches to the anterior and lateral intercondylar eminence of the tibia.

Posterior cruciate ligament –– This originates from the lateral wall of the medial femoral condyle and attaches to the posterior intercondylar eminence of the tibia.

What are the symptoms of a ruptured anterior cruciate ligament?

Immediate swelling of the knee (haemarthrosis), as the ACL is a vascular structure, and inability to bear weight fully. The patient often hears a pop. After injury, symptoms of instability and 'giving way' of the knee occur, and the patient often states that the knee cannot be trusted. Pain is not often a classical symptom of the injury.

How is the anterior cruciate ligament commonly injured?

The ACL is ruptured most commonly in athletes, at the time of pivoting the leg with a lateral rotational movement of the knee. The most common sports that lead to an ACL injury are netball, football and rugby.

What types of graft are used to reconstruct the ACL?

Autologous (hamstrings or patella tendon), allograft (cadaveric) or synthetic material. Autologous grafts are most commonly used, in particular hamstring tendons. Patients can experience weak hamstrings in hamstring grafts, and can develop tendonitis in patella grafts.

What is the O'Donoghue's triad (or unhappy triad, terrible triad)?

It is an injury to the anterior cruciate ligament, medial collateral ligament (MCL) and meniscus (medial or lateral). The original triad described by O'Donoghue stated the medial meniscus but the lateral has been incorporated as it is more commonly seen among athletes with such injuries.

Lumbar vertebrae

What are the five divisions of the spinal column?

- Cervical,
- Thoracic,
- Lumbar,
- Sacrum,
- Coccyx.

How many lumbar vertebrae are usually present?

Five.

What are the characteristic features of the lumbar vertebra?

See Figure 5.9.

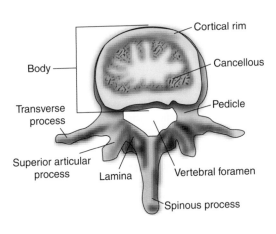

Figure 5.9
Lumbar vertebra (axial view).

- Large vertebral body (lateral plane is wider than the anteroposterior plane).
- Pedicles are very strong and positioned at the posterior end of the vertebral body.
- Superior articular surface is vertical and concave. The facets are positioned backwards and medially, while the inferior articular processes are convex and directed forward and laterally.
- Laminae are broad, short and strong (the lamina connects the pedicles to the spinous process).
- The spinous process that points posteriorly is quadrangular in shape.
- Quadrangular vertebral foramen (larger than the foramen in the thoracic vertebra).
- Absence of foramina in the transverse processes (cf. cervical).
- Absence of costal facets on the side of the body or on the transverse process (cf. thoracic).
- Transverse processes are long and horizontal in the upper three lumbar vertebrae and incline upwards in the lower two vertebrae. They are situated anterior to the articular surface (cf. posterior in the thoracic vertebrae).

What is the term given when the L5 vertebra is fused to the first sacral vertebra?

Sacralization. This is a congenital anomaly; L5 can be fused on one or both sides. This can cause confusion in assessing the radiographs of the lumbar spine. It is best identified by counting down from T12 as opposed to counting up from L5.

What is the term given when the first sacral vertebra has an articulation with the second sacral vertebra?

Lumbarization. This is less common than sacralization: S1 appears like a sixth lumbar vertebra and may have a disc space or a rudimentary disc space.

Which lumbar vertebra is the commonest site of spondylolysis and spondylolisthesis?

The fifth lumbar vertebra.

What structures are attached to the lumbar transverse processes?

Psoas fascia and the origin or psoas muscle before it joins the iliacus to form the iliopsoas. The iliolumbar ligament (from which the quadrates lumborum muscle arises) is attached to the transverse ligament of the fifth vertebra.

What are the intervertebral discs?

They are secondary cartilaginous joints found between pairs of vertebral bodies throughout the vertebral column to allow slight movement of the vertebrae. The intervertebral disc is comprised of the outer or peripheral annulus fibrosus and the central nucleus polposus.

What is their purpose?

With the tough annulus fibrosus, the nucleus polposus acts as a shock absorber absorbing the impact of daily activities. The intervertebral discs also act to separate the vertebrae. However, as people age, the nucleus polposus dehydrates, which limits its ability to absorb axial forces, and the annulus undergoes degenerative tears. These pathological processes can lead to chronic back pain.

In which direction do discs usually prolapse?

The most common prolapse is in the posterolateral direction, as the posterior longitudinal ligament usually prevents a direct posterior prolapse. The former can cause nerve root compression. However, if posterior prolapse occurs, it may cause compression of the cauda equina, which is an orthopaedic emergency.

Popliteal fossa

Where is the popliteal fossa situated and what are its boundaries?

The popliteal fossa (Figure 5.10) is a diamond-shaped area situated in the posterior aspect of the knee.

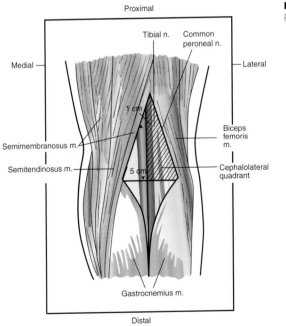

Figure 5.10
Popliteal fossa.

Supra-medial border	Biceps femoris muscle,
Supra-lateral border	Semi-tendinosus and semi-membranosus muscles,
Infra-medial border	Medial head of gastrocnemius muscle,
Infra-lateral border	Lateral head of gastrocnemius muscle,
Floor (deep)	Popliteal surface of the femur, posterior capsule of the knee joint and the oblique popliteal ligament, and the fascia covering the popliteal muscle,
Roof (superficial)	Deep fascia, superficial fascia (containing short saphenous vein, three cutaneous nerves) and skin.

What are the contents of the popliteal fossa?

From deep to superficial (important in any patient with an open injury or laceration in this region):

- Popliteal artery (a continuation of the femoral artery).
- Popliteal vein.
- Tibial and common peroneal nerve (branches of the sciatic nerve – the division could occur anywhere from the sciatic notch to the popliteal fossa). The common peroneal nerve is the most superficial structure, and runs along the supra-lateral border of the fossa, adjacent to the biceps femoris, exiting the fossa at the infra-lateral aspect over the lateral head of gastrocnemius and into and along the peroneus longus.
- Popliteal lymph nodes.
- Short saphenous vein.
- Posterior cutaneous nerve of the thigh.

What clinical aspects are useful with the anatomical knowledge of the popliteal fossa?

- Palpation of the popliteal pulse. This can be difficult, especially in an obese patient, because the artery is the deepest structure. An aid to palpating it is to flex the knee to 30° and palpate the artery against the bony floor.
- Knowledge of the superficial nature of the nerves enables the anaesthetist to deliver a popliteal local anaesthetic block.
- The assessment of neurovascular injuries in any fracture or knee dislocation, especially in high velocity or sporting injuries, is aided.

Radial nerve

From what part of the brachial plexus does the radial nerve branch?

The radial nerve is the largest branch of the posterior cord of the brachial plexus (nerve roots C5–T1).

Describe the course of the radial nerve in the arm

The radial nerve runs from its origin as a continuation of the posterior cord of the brachial plexus exiting the axilla into the posterior compartment of the arm along the posterior aspect of the axillary artery through the triangular space bordered by the long head of triceps, the humerus and the teres major.

Along its path, the radial nerve gives off motor branches to the long and medial heads of the triceps, and the posterior cutaneous nerve of the arm (sensory). It lies in the spiral groove of the humerus, giving off branches to the lateral head of triceps and anconeus, as well as the posterior cutaneous nerve of the forearm distally.

The radial nerve exits the posterior compartment through the lateral intramuscular septum and into the cubital fossa. This is where it divides into its two terminal branches; the (predominantly sensory) radial nerve and the (predominantly motor) posterior interosseous nerve (PIN).

The PIN enters and supplies the extensor compartment of the forearm, travelling around the proximal radius and through the supinator.

The radial nerve continues within the forearm under the brachioradialis. It travels briefly along with and medial to the radial artery. It eventually pierces the deep fascia posteriorly and supplies the skin at the dorsal aspect of the wrist and hand.

At what site is the radial nerve commonly injured?

It is injured at the spiral groove of the humerus in humeral fractures (middle third) and its fixation, and at the axilla, secondary to traction injuries from shoulder dislocations, 'axilla' crutches, or 'Saturday night palsy' (these traction injuries are usually temporary – neuropraxia).

The posterior interosseous nerve can be injured from proximal radial fractures.

What are the clinical presentations of radial nerve injuries in the various areas along its route?

At the axilla –– Leads to paralysis of triceps and the forearm and wrist extensors. This gives loss of extension in the elbow, wrist and hand with unopposed flexors – wrist drop. Loss of sensation is most pronounced over the dorsum of the hand.

At the distal humerus or spiral groove –– Wrist drop, as above.

At the proximal radius –– Injury to the posterior interosseous nerve causing loss of finger extension without a wrist drop. Extensor carpi radialis (and brachialis) function are preserved, as they are supplied by the main radial nerve. The PIN is a motor nerve.

How would you test for the radial nerve?

Motor function is tested by the power of wrist dorsiflexion and finger extension (to include the posterior interosseous nerve).

Sensory function is tested in the autonomous sensory area of the radial nerve, which is over the dorsal aspect of the first web space.

Sciatic nerve

Where is the greater sciatic foramen?

The greater sciatic foramen is situated in the pelvis between the greater sciatic notch and both the sacrospinous and sacrotuberous ligaments.

What passes through it?

Various structures pass through the foramen. The major structures include:

- Piriformis muscle (lateral rotator of the hip),
- Sciatic nerve,
- Superior and inferior gluteal nerves,
- Pudendal nerve,
- Superior and inferior gluteal vessels.

What are the surface markings of the sciatic nerve?

The sciatic nerve lies in the medial and posterior (lower, inner) quadrant of the buttock and travels inferiorly midway between the ischial tuberosity and the greater trochanter of the femur. It runs vertically initially deep to the gluteus maximus, then down the midline of the posterior compartment of the thigh until its bifurcation into the tibial and common peroneal nerves (usually two-thirds of the way down). Superiorly, it is in close proximity to the posterior rim of the acetabulum. This needs to be considered, especially in the posterior approach to the hip during total hip replacement.

Where would you give buttock intramuscular injections?

They should be given in the supra-lateral (upper, outer) quadrant of the buttock to avoid the sciatic nerve, which lies in the medial posterior quadrant.

What are the nerve roots of the sciatic nerve?

The anterior primary rami of L4, L5, S1, S2, and S3.

What are the branches of the sciatic nerve and where does it divide?

The sciatic nerve divides into the tibial and common peroneal nerves. Division can occur anywhere from the sciatic notch to the popliteal fossa (most commonly two-thirds of the way down the thigh).

Note that the sciatic nerve gives off a branch to the posterior compartment of the thigh supplying some of the short lateral rotators of the hip and the hamstrings.

What motor deficits are seen in a sciatic nerve injury?

- If the injury is proximal to the knee, loss of hamstring function occurs.
- If the injury is distal to the knee joint, loss of function in all the leg muscles and the patient will produce a foot drop.

What sensory deficits are seen in a sciatic nerve injury?

Loss of sensation below the knee. The saphenous nerve is a sensory nerve and a branch of the femoral nerve and therefore the areas supplied by the saphenous nerve are spared. This includes the medial aspect of the leg, medial side of the ankle and up to the mid foot (some crossover exists between the nerves).

Shoulder

What type of joint is the shoulder joint and what joint does it correspond to in the lower limb?

The shoulder joint (Figure 5.11) is a synovial ball-and-socket joint between the humeral head (with the articular surface facing medially) and the glenoid. It corresponds to the hip joint, which is another ball-and-socket joint.

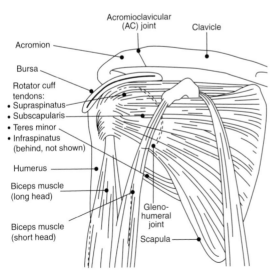

Figure 5.11
Shoulder.

Is the shoulder joint seen to be intrinsically stable or unstable?

Unstable.

What structures around the glenohumeral joint augment its stability?

Muscles	Rotator cuff muscles (supraspinatus, infraspinatus, teres minor, subscapularis).
Ligaments	Glenohumeral, coracohumeral, coracoacromial.
Tendons	Long head of biceps and tendon of triceps.
Capsule	Weakest inferiorly.
Glenoid labrum	As with the labrum in the hip, this increases the depth of the 'socket' and aids stability.

What muscles insert to the greater tuberosity and the proximal humerus?

Greater tuberosity	Supraspinatus, infraspinatus and teres minor,
Proximal humerus	Pectoralis major, latissimus dorsi and teres minor.

What muscles are attached to the coracoid process?

The short head of the biceps and the coracobrachialis originate at the coracoid process, and the pectoralis minor attaches to it.

What is the role of the bursae around the shoulder?

They permit smooth gliding of the rotator cuff muscles, and protect them from the bony arches of the acromion.

What is the most common shoulder dislocation?

- Anterior dislocations account for around 95% of shoulder dislocations. The mechanism is usually a fall onto an outstretched hand or a direct trauma onto the shoulder, where the humeral head goes into abduction and externally rotates out of the joint, leaving the arm clinically held in an abducted, externally rotated position. The resultant position of the humeral head is anterior to the scapula.

- Posterior dislocations account for the remaining 5%. This type of dislocation is most commonly associated with epileptic fits and electrocutions. These injuries are also more commonly missed, leading to significant morbidity.

What associated injuries are seen with shoulder dislocations?

Rotator cuff injury including tears, bony injury to the articular surface of the humeral head (Hill-Sachs lesion), or injury to the glenoid labrum (Bankart lesion).

What nerve injury can occur with an anterior dislocation, what does it supply and how is it tested?

An injury to the axillary nerve. This causes paralysis of the deltoid muscle, which leads to inability to abduct the shoulder. To test whether this nerve is intact, sensation is tested over the 'regimental badge area' across the proximal lateral aspect of the arm. This, as well as distal pulses, needs to be clearly documented in any patient with a shoulder dislocation, pre- and post-reduction.

Spinal cord

Describe the internal structure of the spinal cord

- The spinal cord (Figure 5.12) consists of grey and white matter.
- The grey matter is found centrally and is arranged in a 'butterfly' shape. It is organized as ten laminae on each side, containing sensory and motor nerve cells:

Laminae I–VI	Receive cutaneous and visceral primary afferent fibres,
Laminae VII, VIII and X	Centrally positioned and receive no peripheral fibres,
Laminae IX	Lies in the anterior horn and contains α and γ motoneurons.

- The white matter contains the ascending and descending tracts.

Ascending tracts (sensory)

Dorsal columns	Deep touch, fine tactile, proprioception, vibration,
Lateral spinothalamic	Pain, temperature, tactile sense,
Anterior spinothalamic	Light touch,
Spinocerebellar	Proprioception

Descending tracts (motor)

Lateral corticospinal	Skilled voluntary movements,
Anterior corticospinal	Voluntary control,
Vestibulospinal and reticulospinal	Controls tone and posture.

Note: the corticospinal tract is the main motor descending tract and is also known as the *pyramidal tract*. The other (vestibulospinal and reticulospinal) tracts constitute the *extrapyramidal* tract.

Where do motor pathways decussate?

The descending corticospinal tracts decussate as they exit the medulla and travel down the cord on the contralateral side.

Where do sensory pathways decussate?

The ascending spinothalamic tract decussates obliquely in the cord before ascending.

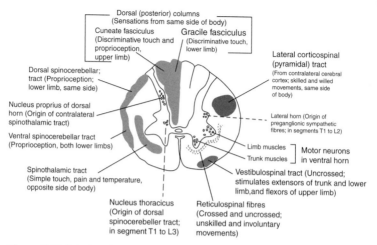

Figure 5.12 Spinal cord.

Spinal cord: blood supply

What three major arteries run the length of the spinal cord?

Blood to the vertebral column and the spinal cord is supplied by several segmental arteries that arise from the aorta and nearby arteries. The three major arteries that supply the cord are:

- Two posterior spinal arteries lying around the posterolateral sulci,
- An anterior spinal artery running in the ventral midline from foramen magnum to the filum terminale.

These three arteries anastomose around the spinal cord and supply it.

Which of these arteries is considered the predominant supply to the cord?

The anterior spinal artery. It is supplied by 4–10 large unpaired medullary or radicular arteries that originate from vertebral arteries and the aorta (often one to the cervical, two to the thoracic and one to the lumbar cord). It supplies the anterior two-thirds of the spinal cord, including most of the grey matter.

What is the artery of Adamkiewicz?

This artery, which has many variations, is a single medullary artery positioned usually on the left of the aorta (around T10–T12), supplying the thoracolumbar cord via the anterior spinal artery.

What are the consequences of injury or damage to the artery of Adamkiewicz?

This could lead to cord ischaemia and paralysis from an anterior cord syndrome.

Does the posterior spinal artery have any equivalent large branches, such as the artery of Adamkiewicz?

No. The posterior spinal artery receives 30–40 smaller medullary tributaries, but none is as large as the anterior branches.

Where are the veins of the spinal cord located?

They are in the pia mater, where they form a plexus. They drain into the internal vertebral venous plexuses, which are located between the dura and the vertebrae within the vertebral canal.

Chapter 6

Operative surgery

Carpal tunnel decompression

What are the causes of carpal tunnel syndrome?

Any condition that increases the pressure within the carpal tunnel will lead to compression of the median nerve and thus symptoms of median nerve entrapment. These conditions include:

- Pregnancy,
- Hypothyroidism,
- Acromegaly,
- Rheumatoid arthritis,
- Trauma: this can occur as a complication of a Colles' fracture.

How would you perform a carpal tunnel decompression?

- Obtain informed consent from the patient.
- Mark the arm with a permanent marker.
- Apply tourniquet and infiltrate with local anaesthetic.
- Have the arm laid out onto arm board, supinated, prepared and draped.
- Consider using a 'lead hand retractor' to expose the hand and keep it flat.
- Make an incision in line with the third web space, beginning approximately 3 cm distal to the distal wrist crease.
- The incision should not cross the distal wrist crease, to avoid painful scarring.
- Ensure that the incision is perpendicular to the skin at all times.
- A West self-retaining retractor is useful for visualizing the retinaculum as the dissection progresses.
- The median nerve is protected by sliding a MacDonald's elevator immediately beneath the retinaculum.
- The retinaculum is then incised until the palmar arch and the visualization of the palmar fat pad.

- Ensure that the retinaculum is released proximally.
- Achieve haemostasis.
- Close the skin with interrupted nylon sutures.
- Apply dressing and bandages.

What nerves are at risk in this procedure?

Median nerve

Palmar cutaneous branch of the median nerve	Passes superficial to the flexor retinaculum on the radial side of palmaris longus and is the sensory supply to the thenar eminence,
Recurrent motor branch of the median nerve	Branches radially as the median nerve exits the carpal tunnel, and turns back to give the motor supply the thenar muscles.
Ulnar nerve and ulnar artery	If the dissection goes towards the ulnar aspect and into Guyon's canal – thus the emphasis on a straight incision with perpendicular dissection.

Where is the ulnar nerve and is it affected by a carpal tunnel syndrome?

No, the ulnar nerve is not affected in a carpal tunnel syndrome. The ulnar nerve and ulnar artery run on the ulnar aspect of the flexor retinaculum in their own tunnel, called Guyon's canal. The ulnar nerve can sustain similar compression symptoms, but is relatively rare.

Colles' fracture reduction

What is a Colles' fracture?

This is an extra-articular distal radius fracture (Figure 6.1), which is described as a 'dinner-fork' deformity. It includes shortening of the distal radial height, dorsal angulation and displacement of the distal fragment and radial angulation and displacement.

How do you perform a closed reduction of the Colles' fracture?

- Obtain informed consent.
- Under aseptic conditions, administer a haematoma block with lignocaine and Marcaine (bupivacaine), for a longer anaesthetic effect. The aim is to insert the needle into the fracture site. While performing a haematoma block, await for 'flash-back' of blood from the fracture haematoma prior to injection. This should have the colour of dark venous blood.
- Apply longitudinal traction (to achieve relaxation of the antagonist muscles) with an assistant providing counter traction (above the elbow)

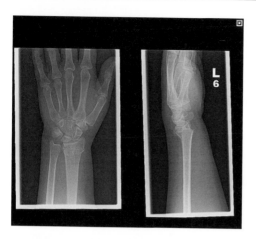

Figure 6.1 X-ray of Colles' fracture showing dorsal angulation of an extra-articular distal radial fracture.

while the surgeon controls the distal fragment and wrist with both hands. Beware of the force applied as this might cause a degloving injury in the frail, the elderly or patients on steroid medication. The force should not exceed the surgeon's and assistant's body weight.

- Traction should be followed by hyperextension of the distal fragment to disengage it from the fracture, then translate it distally (while in extended position) until it can be 'hooked over' the proximal fragment.

- The distal fragment should then be flexed to hinge it on the proximal shaft fragment and achieve realignment.

- Maintaining traction, the fracture should have some stability in its reduced position.

- The wrist should be now held in a slight palmar flexion and ulnar deviation while plaster of Paris is applied.

- In the acute stages, this should allow for swelling of the forearm, therefore a 'tram line' or back-slab should be applied.

- Postreduction X-rays should be obtained to ensure satisfactory alignment of the fracture fragments.

- Follow-up should be within one week with a repeat X-ray to ensure no displacement has occurred and re-enforcement or completion of the cast should be carried out.

What are the late complications of a Colles' fracture?

- Malunion if the fragments have slipped from their point of reduction (malunion is much more common than non-union): this has the consequence of limitation of wrist movements.

- Carpal tunnel syndrome: tension, swelling and occasionally bony fragments from the volar aspect could apply pressure on the median nerve and cause symptoms of carpal tunnel syndrome. Patients should be assessed for carpal tunnel syndrome prereduction. If symptoms do not resolve, a formal carpal tunnel decompression will be required.
- Tendon rupture: most commonly, the extensor pollicis longus (EPL).

Compartment syndrome and fasciotomy

What is compartment syndrome?

Compartment syndrome occurs in the presence of raised pressure in an enclosed fixed space, such as an osseofascial compartment, exceeding perfusion pressure and compromising the circulation and function of the tissues within the compartment. It reduces capillary flow as well as venous return, leading to venous congestion and oedema, until such pressure compromises the arterial supply to the compartment contents. The effect of this is temporary or permanent ischaemia to the muscles and nerves, which also contributes to furthering the oedema and pressure rise.

Where is compartment syndrome most commonly seen?

In the lower limb, specifically the leg, which has four compartments: anterior, lateral, superficial and deep posterior. The anterior compartment (the extensors) are most commonly affected, leading to loss of hallux and toe extension as well as loss of dorsiflexion from the effect on the tibialis anterior.

The foot and forearm have several compartments each.

What are the causes of compartment syndrome?

Internal causes
- Fractures: high energy closed injuries or open injuries,
- Haemorrhage: trauma, anticoagulation, postoperative procedures on limb,
- Crush injury,
- Burns,
- Insect or snake bites,
- Rhabdomyolysis.

External causes
- Burns,
- Tight casts or splints,
- Any external localized pressure or garment restriction.

How is compartment syndrome diagnosed?

Whenever compartment syndrome is suspected, urgent action is needed, as this is an orthopaedic emergency. The history of the method of injury is key.

- Pain is out of proportion of the physical signs and increasing in nature and uncontrolled with analgesia,
- Passive starching of the affected muscles causing severe pain,
- Paraesthesia,
- Paralysis, pulselessness and pallor are late signs,
- Measurement of intra-compartmental pressure (can be done at the bedside) using a transducer or a needle attached to a manometer: indicative pressure would be a single reading >40 mmHg, persistent reading of 30 mmHg for over four hours or >20 mmHg greater than the normal contralateral leg.

How would you treat compartment syndrome of the leg?

- This is a surgical emergency.
- Split and remove cast or plaster and bandages (if present) down to skin to assess the limb further.
- The patient needs to be prepared for theatre, for urgent fasciotomy of all involved compartments.
- Use a double longitudinal incision technique (Figure 6.2) 2 cm from the anteromedial and anterolateral border of the tibia (the former to preserve the perforators at 5, 10 and 15 cm, to allow for distally based fasciocutaneous flaps).[1]
- Decompress the superficial and deep compartments through the medial longitudinal incision and the lateral and anterior compartments though the lateral longitudinal incision.
- Leave open and revisit in 48 hours for inspection, debridement and primary delayed closure, with or without skin grafting.

Fractured neck of femur

What is the blood supply to the femoral head?

There are three main sources:

Interosseous nutrient artery	Via the medullary canal of the femur.
Ligamentum teres	The artery found at the fovea of the femoral head. It is considered more

---

[1] www.boa.ac.uk/en/publications/boast/.

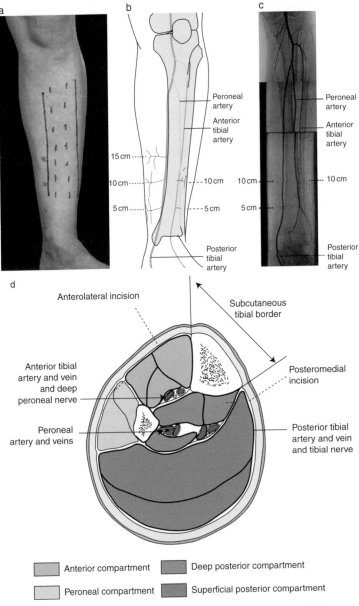

Figure 6.2 (a) Marking the leg to show margins of subcutaneous border of tibia, fasciotomy incisions and the perforators on the medial side arising from the posterior tibial vessels. (b) Location of perforators. (c) Arteriogram to show disruption of anterior tibial artery following open dislocation of ankle. (d) Cross-section through the leg showing incisions to decompress all four compartments. (BOA and BARAS Guidelines, 2009).

| Retinacular vessels from the trochanteric anastomosis | important in contributing to the blood supply in children and infants. |
| | The medial and lateral circumflex arteries (branches of profunda femoris), which travel within the joint capsule and are reflected back towards the head at the capsular attachment to the femur. Disruption of these vessels is assumed in intracapsular fractures, thus dictating management. |

What is the commonly used classification of femoral neck fractures?

- The most common way to describe a neck of femur fracture is in relation to the capsule: intracapsular or extracapsular.
- This is helpful in dictating the type of procedure needed; whether it is a hemiarthroplasty, total hip replacement, cannulated screws or dynamic hip screw fixation.

What is Garden's classification?

This a classification of fractures of the intracapsular neck of the femur, based on the displacement of the fracture evident on an anteroposterior hip radiograph. See Figure 6.3.

I   Incomplete or impacted,
II   Complete and undisplaced,
III Complete with partial displacement,
IV   Complete with full displacement.

What is the significance of the classification and how does it relate to treatment?

The aim is always to preserve the patient's femoral head, if possible. All intracapsular fractures carry a risk of disrupting the blood supply to the femoral head and thus increasing the rate of avascular necrosis. The Garden grades correlate with the prognosis and increased risk of femoral head osteonecrosis. The common method of fixation of grades I and II is with a 'screw' (this can be done using cannulated screws or dynamic hip screw (DHS) since the blood supply is likely to be intact, in contrast with III and IV). This should be done as soon as possible after injury, ideally within six hours. Grades III and IV are usually treated with a hemiarthroplasty (cemented or uncemented), or a total hip replacement if the patient is relatively young or active.

While performing the screw fixation (DHS or cannulated screws), in what position are you aiming to place your guidewire?

The aim is to get the guidewire at the centre of the femoral head in both the anteroposterior (AP) and lateral plane on the image intensifier (II).

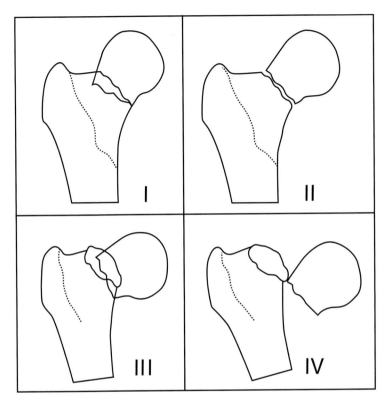

Figure 6.3 Fractures to the neck of the femur.

The unfavourable positions, which increase the risk of cutting out of the screw and failure of the fixation, are those where the screw is placed too superior or too anterior or posterior. The tip–apex distance (TAD), which is the distance between the centre of the femoral head and the tip of the screw in both the anteroposterior and lateral planes, when combined, should not exceed 25 mm.

What should the weight-bearing status of the patient be immediately after the operation?

The patient should be fully weight-bearing with the assistance of physiotherapists, unless there were specific intra-operative complications that prohibit this. This will decrease the risk of developing a deep vein thrombosis.

If the fracture were below the lesser trochanter (i.e. subtrochanteric), what other type of prosthesis would you consider?

An intramedullary nail (a long nail with a hip screw fixation).

With what other configuration of an extracapsular neck-of-femur fracture would you consider the above device, and why?

Reverse oblique fractures, owing to the loss of the lateral wall and increased stability provided.

What are the complications seen with extracapsular neck-of-femur fractures or intracapsular fractures that are fixed with screws?

- Avascular necrosis,
- Malunion or non-union,
- Progression of osteoarthritis,
- General complications, including infection, neurovascular injury, deep vein thromboses, pulmonary embolisms, decreased mobility, urinary tract infections, chest infection and pressure sores.

In an elderly patient, this could be a life-threatening event. Mortality rates for inpatients are as high as 10–15%. Mortality in the first year is around 33%.

Management of open fractures

What is considered an open fracture?

An open fracture is defined as a fracture that has breached the skin and is in communication with the outside environment. The size of the communication can vary from a puncture wound in the skin to a large avulsion of soft tissue that leaves the bone exposed.

What is the primary management of open fractures? (from 2009 BOA & BAPRAS guidelines)

- Initial assessment of the patient should occur simultaneously, under ATLS principles.
- Re-assess the open fracture (commonly tibial), to establish any evolving limb-threatening conditions.
- Control haemorrhaging through direct pressure or, as a last resort, application of a tourniquet.
- Wounds must only be handled to remove gross contaminants, for photography or to seal them from the environment.
- Wounds should not be explored or irrigated in the emergency department.
- Immobilize the limb with any type of splint available – usually plaster of Paris.

- Administer intravenous antibiotics. This should be done as soon after the injury as possible and within three hours. The antibiotic of choice is co-amoxiclav (1.2 g every eight hours), or a cephalosporin (e.g. cefuroxime 1.5 g every eight hours), and this should be continued for at least 72 hours or until soft-tissue closure. Add metronidazole if the wound has been in contact with farmyard manure or sewage.
- Determine anti-tetanus status and give tetanus booster if indicated.
- Take anteroposterior and lateral X-ray of the fractured limb with X-rays of the joint above and below.

What are the reasons for immediate surgical exploration?

- Gross contamination of the wound,
- Compartment syndrome,
- A de-vascularized limb,
- A multiply injured patient.

Otherwise, soft tissue and bone excision (debridement) should be performed by senior plastic or orthopaedic surgeons on a scheduled trauma list within normal working hours but within 24 hours of the injury, unless there is marine, agricultural or sewage contamination. The six-hour rule does not apply for solitary open fractures.

What are the general guidelines for wound debridement?

- Early, accurate debridement of the traumatic wound is the most important surgical procedure in the management of open tibial fractures. Debridement means excision of all devitalized tissue.
- Traumatic wounds are excised comprehensively and systematically. This can be done under tourniquet, but if used it needs to be deflated at the time of bone debridement to ensure bone bleeding of remaining fragments.
- Initially, the limb is washed with a soapy solution and then prepared with an alcoholic chlorhexidine solution, avoiding contact of the antiseptic with the open wound.
- The tissues are assessed systematically in turn, from superficial to deep (skin, fat, muscle, bone) and from the periphery to the centre of the wound. Non-viable skin, fat, muscle and bone are excised. Loose fragments of bone that fail the 'tug test' are removed.
- Continuous irrigation should be used to clear the visibility of the surgical field, but high-pressure pulsatile lavage is not recommended, as it can propagate contamination deeper into the tissues.

- At this stage, the injury can be classified and definitive reconstruction planned jointly by the senior members of the orthopaedic and plastic surgical team.
- Vacuum dressing can be applied in two-stage procedures, if the wounds remain open due to delayed reconstruction.

What is the Gustilo and Anderson classification system[2] for open fractures?

Type I   Clean wound smaller than 1 cm in diameter; appears clean, simple fracture pattern, no skin crushing.

Type II   A laceration larger than 1 cm but without significant soft-tissue crushing, including no flaps, degloving or contusion. Fracture pattern may be more complex.

Type III   An open segmental fracture or a single fracture with extensive soft-tissue injury. Also included are injuries older than eight hours.

Type III injuries are subdivided into three subtypes:

Type IIIA   Adequate soft tissue coverage of the fracture despite high energy trauma or extensive laceration or skin flaps.

Type IIIB   Inadequate soft tissue coverage with periosteal stripping. Soft tissue reconstruction is necessary.

Type IIIC   Any open fracture that is associated with vascular injury that requires repair.

What is the prognosis of each type of open fracture in terms of expected rate of infection and risk of amputation?

Gustilo type I   Infection rate 0%; amputation rate 0–2%,

Gustilo type II   Infection rate 0%; amputation rate 2–7%,

Gustilo type IIIA   Infection rate 7%; amputation rate 2.5%,

Gustilo type IIIB   Infection rate 10–50%; amputation rate 5%,

Gustilo type IIIC   Infection rate 25–50%; amputation rate 25%.

What are the limitations of the Gustilo and Anderson classification system?

It has poor interobserver reliability. It is best utilized after wound excision.

What are the complications of open fractures?

- Acute wound infection, which can lead to osteomyelitis, chronic osteomyelitis and possibly amputation.

---

[2] R. B. Gustilo and J. T. Anderson (1976) Prevention of infection in the treatment of one thousand and twenty-five open fractures of long bones: retrospective and prospective analyses. *J. Bone Joint Surg. Am.* **58**:453–8.

- Infection rates vary (as mentioned) but the likelihood of infection also depends on the degree of associated soft-tissue injury and the initial management of the patient. Infections may result from pathogens at the time of injury or may be acquired in the hospital.
- Infection can lead to delayed healing or non-union.
- There is a risk of tetanus infection, especially if the patient has not been vaccinated.
- Neurovascular injury is more common in type III injuries.
- Compartment syndrome may develop.

Principles of amputation

What are the indications for amputation of a limb?

- Peripheral vascular disease (acute ischaemia),
- Trauma:
  - Insensate limb distally,
  - Unsalvageable limb.
- Infection (especially necrotizing fasciitis, gangrene),
- Tumours,
- Nerve injury (trophic ulceration),
- Congenital anomalies.

What are the general aims when amputating any limb?

- Return to maximum level of independent function,
- Removal of diseased tissue,
- Reduce morbidity and mortality,
- Requires a multidisciplinary approach.

What is the optimum amputation level for prosthesis fitting in above and below knee amputations?

Table 6.1 Optimum amputation levels

Amputation levels	Optimum	Shortest	Longest
Above knee	Middle third	8 cm below pubic ramus	15 cm above medial joint line of knee
Below knee	8 cm for every metre of height	7.5 cm below medial joint line of knee	Level at which myoplasty is possible

What precautions do you need to be aware of in the closure of the skin of the amputation stump?

- Do not close skin under tension.
- Interrupted sutures are advisable.

What are the complications of amputation?

- Haematoma,
- Wound complications: infection or dehiscence,
- Skin necrosis and distal ischaemia,
- Oedema,
- Contractures,
- Neuroma,
- Phantom pain,
- Terminal overgrowth (children).

What are the contraindications to a below-knee amputation?

- Severe osteoarthritis in the knee,
- Significant joint contractures,
- Ischaemia at the level of amputation (therefore will require a higher amputation),
- Infection at the level of amputation (therefore will require a higher amputation),
- Neuropathy at the level of amputation.

Principles of arthroscopy

What is arthroscopic surgery?

This is a minimally invasive surgical procedure, where an arthroscope (a type of endoscope) is inserted into the joint through small 'keyhole' incisions, for the purpose of examination and treatment of the joint.

What are the advantages of arthroscopy vs. open surgery?

- The joint is not opened; there are only two small incisions for the portals to introduce an arthroscope and surgical instruments,
- Reduced recovery time,
- Less trauma to connective tissue,
- Less scarring,
- Decreased rate of infection than for the same procedures done using the open technique.

What are the specific complications of arthroscopic surgery?

- Fluid used to distend the joint can extravasate into surrounding tissues, causing oedema and, rarely, compartment syndrome.
- Portal site pain.
- Iatrogenic chondral injury caused by the trocar introducer, or iatrogenic meniscal injury while making the incision of portals.

What are the two common portals used in knee arthroscopy?

- Anterolateral portal (usually for the arthroscope),
- Anteromedial portal (usually made under direct vision).

What common conditions can be treated and assessed using knee arthroscopy?

- Meniscal tears,
- Reconstructions of the anterior and posterior cruciate ligaments,
- Osteochondral flaps,
- Osteochondral defects treated with microfractures,
- Osteoarthritis, although this is controversial and has limited benefit.

Surgical approaches to the hip

What are the most common approaches to the hip and what are they used for?

Anterolateral (Hardinge) approach –– This is the most common approach used for total hip replacement and hemiarthroplasty. It involves a release of the abductors. It combines an excellent exposure to the acetabulum with safety during reaming of the femoral shaft.

Its uses include: total hip replacement (THR), revision THR, hemiarthroplasty, open reduction and internal fixation (ORIF) of femoral neck fractures, synovial biopsy of the hip and biopsy of the femoral neck.

Posterior approach –– This allows easy, safe and quick access to the joint. As it does not interfere with the abductor mechanism, it does not affect the abductor power postoperatively. It also allows excellent visualization of the femoral shaft. However, there is a theoretical increased risk of hip dislocation following joint replacement due to the disruption of the posterior capsule and the short rotators of the hip (now seen to be equal to other approaches if done correctly).

Its uses include: hemiarthroplasty, THR and revision THR, open reduction and internal fixation (ORIF) of posterior acetabular fractures, and drainage of hip sepsis.

Anterior (Smith-Petersen) approach –– This provides safe access to the hip joint and ilium. It is a common approach in the paediatric hip.

Its uses include: open reduction of congenital hip dislocations, synovial biopsies, paediatric hip wash-out, THR, hemiarthroplasty and excision of pelvic tumours. It can also be used for pelvic osteotomies when used more proximally.

What nerves can be damaged in each of these approaches?

Anterolateral   Inferior branch of superior gluteal nerve,

Posterior   Sciatic nerve,

Anterior   Lateral femoral cutaneous nerve of the thigh.

Describe the anterolateral (Hardinge) approach for a hemiarthroplasty procedure

- The patient is usually placed in the lateral position.
- Skin is incised in a curve starting a hands-breadth distal to the greater trochanter.
- The tensor fascia lata is incised and the gluteus medius tendon is divided, leaving the posterior half or third attached to the greater trochanter. The gluteus minimus is sometimes taken with it or as a separate layer.
- The capsule is then met and either an incision is made (T-shape capsulotomy) or a capsulectomy is performed.
- The femoral neck is then cut using a power saw in line with a femoral stem trial (this can be marked using diathermy). This is best done with the leg in external rotation, which will also ease the extraction of the head once cut.
- The head is then sized and a prosthesis requested – if necessary, it is advisable to round down the head size and not up.
- The femoral stem is then prepared with a box chisel and rasped sequentially.
- The stem is then washed out and cement restrictor is placed in the distal end of the canal, roughly 1 cm distal to the tip of the prosthesis, to receive the antibiotic impregnated cement mantle. If an uncemented prosthesis is planned, this step is skipped.
- The hemiarthroplasty is pressured and hammered in until it is sitting in stable manner onto the calcar femorale.
- The hip is then reduced, checking stability in all planes, and accurate and adequate repair of the abductors to avoid a Trendelenburg's gait.
- Layered closure is used, with an absorbable suture (Vicryl) up to the skin (clips, staples, nylon, Monocryl).

What should the weight-bearing status of the patient be immediately after the operation?

The patient should be fully weight-bearing with the assistance of physiotherapists, unless there were specific intra-operative complications that prohibit this. This will decrease the risk of developing a deep vein thrombosis.

What complications are seen with hip hemiarthroplasty?

- Dislocation (which could lead to sciatic nerve injury leading to a foot drop),
- Leg length discrepancy,
- Peri-prosthetic fracture,
- Infection or loosening of the prosthesis,
- Migration of the prosthesis and erosion of the acetabulum,
- General complications, including infection, neurovascular injury (specifically the sciatic nerve – more so using the posterior approach), deep vein thrombosis or pulmonary embolism, decreased mobility, urinary tract infection, chest infection, pressure sores.

In an elderly patient, this could be a life-threatening event. Mortality rates for inpatients are as high as 10–15%. Mortality in the first year is around 33%.

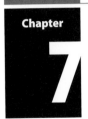

Chapter

7

Clinical examinations (trauma and orthopaedics)

Principles of orthopaedic examination

For any orthopaedic examination, distinct steps should be followed to cover all clinical aspects required in performing an adequate examination and reach a reasonable differential diagnosis:

Inspection

Skin
- Colour – any discolouration of the skin or bruising,
- Abnormal skin creases,
- Scars – surgical vs. non-surgical,
- Sinuses – any visible discharge.

Shape
- Swelling – localized or diffuse; within joint (synovial effusion, haemarthrosis, pyarthrosis) or extending beyond the joint (infections, tumours, lymphatic or venous drainage disruptions),
- Deformity – soft tissue or bone,
- Oedema,
- Muscle wasting – due to inactivity or denervation,
- Lumps – soft tissue or bone,
- Posture or position of limb,
- Shortening.

Gait -- This could be inspected at the beginning or end of the examination, as appropriate. Usually in an examination, the patient is already in the room lying on the couch and therefore, gait would be either examined or discussed at the end of the clinical examination of the specific joint.

Palpation

Skin
- Temperature – localized or diffuse; comparison with normal side is essential (use back of hand),
- Texture of skin,
- Tenderness – localized or diffuse; comparison is crucial, as some sites are tender in normal circumstances.

Soft tissues
- Swelling – localized or diffuse: shape, size, position, consistency, fluctuation,
- Soft tissue masses,
- Tenderness,
- Capsular or synovial thickening,
- Fluid in joint or bursa.

Bones
- Landmarks,
- Tenderness,
- Misalignment,
- Lumps – single or multiple,
- Length of bone – in real and apparent terms.

Movement

Always compare movement with the good side.
- Range of movement: passive and active (as approach to the joint):
  - Flexion,
  - Extension and any fixed flexion deformity,
  - Abduction,
  - Adduction,
  - Internal rotation,
  - External rotation.
- Pain,
- Laxity,
- Crepitus,
- Clicks,
- Mechanical locking.

Special tests

These should be selected according to the joint and the condition being investigated.

Neurovascular examination

- Tone,
- Power – MRC scale M0–M5,
- Sensation,
- Reflexes,
- Coordination,
- Pulses.

Radiology –– Anteroposterior and lateral radiographs of the joint in question (oblique if examining the hand and foot). Other radiographic examinations can be requested depending on the condition, such as ultrasound, CT, MRI, bone scan or white-cell labelled bone scan.

Common adult orthopaedic injuries

A brief description of common orthopaedic injuries and the common mode of treatment.

Shoulder dislocation

Anterior –– This is the most common (95%). The brachial plexus, axillary artery and nerve are at risk of injury. Patients present with pain, deformity with loss of the normal shoulder contour, and holding the arm in slight abduction and external rotation with inability to touch their contralateral shoulder.

Treatment –– Reduction under analgesia or sedation in the emergency department or under general anaesthesia in theatre if necessary. X-rays before and after reduction should be taken and vigilance in detecting the presence of a fracture. Treat with a sling and physiotherapy. Recurrent dislocation might warrant surgical repair of the rotator cuff.

Posterior –– This is rare (5%). It is seen in patients after a seizure or electrocution. The brachial plexus, axillary artery and nerve are at risk of injury. Posterior dislocations are more difficult to detect clinically and on X-rays than anterior dislocations. Patients usually present with arm in slight adduction and internal rotation.

Treatment –– Treatment is the same as for anterior dislocations.

Humeral fracture

This is usually the result of a direct trauma. Proximal humeral fractures at the surgical neck are common in osteoporotic patients. In diaphyseal and distant fractures, the radial nerve always needs to be tested, as it runs along the distal aspect of the humerus against bone. Radial nerve palsy leads to wrist drop (loss of wrist extension) and decrease in sensation over the dorsum of the first web space.

Treatment -- The treatment depends on the configuration of the fracture, the part of the humerus fractured (proximal, midshaft, distal, intra-articular) and the age of the patient. Options include non-operative treatment using a collar and cuff, a sling, hanging arm cast or a functional brace. Operative treatment includes intramedullary nail and open reduction internal fixation (ORIF) with plate and screws.

Monteggia's fracture

This is a fracture of the proximal ulna with dislocation of the radial head.

Treatment -- Treatment is by closed reduction of the radial head. The fracture may then be treated in a cast but commonly needs open reduction internal fixation (ORIF) of the proximal ulna if there is displacement.

Galeazzi's fracture

This is a fracture of the radius (classically the distal to middle third) with dislocation or subluxation of the distal radioulnar joint.

Treatment -- In children, an attempt at closed reduction should be made; however, this injury is usually treated operatively with open reduction and internal fixation (especially in adults).

Colles' fracture

This is a common orthopaedic injury seen in elderly (osteoporotic) patients, after a fall onto the outstretched hand, leading to a fracture of the distal radius with dorsal angulation and loss of radial height. This is an extra-articular fracture of the wrist.

Treatment -- Closed manipulation should be attempted, to restore the length and angulation of the fracture, with a well-moulded plaster of Paris cast. Alternatively, if this fails, operative fixation using K-wires, plate and screw, or external fixation should be attempted.

Night-stick fracture

This is caused after a direct trauma to the ulna shaft or distal third of the ulna after using the forearm for self-defence to block a blow. It is considered unstable if it is displaced >50% with 10° angulation. Monteggia-type fractures need to be ruled out.

Treatment -- Night-stick fractures can be treated in a cast if considered stable, otherwise open reduction internal fixation is required.

Scaphoid fracture

This is the most common fracture of the carpal bones, usually occurring in young adults. Evidence on radiographs can take up to two weeks to appear. The history usually includes falling onto the outstretched hand and examination reveals tenderness in the anatomical snuffbox. Non-union is a common complication, as is avascular necrosis, which occurs in the proximal pole of the scaphoid owing to its blood supply from distal to proximal (see pp. 89–90).

Treatment –– This should be instigated if tenderness in the anatomical snuffbox is present. It should be treated with a thumb spica plaster of Paris cast – but if there is displacement or evidence on non-union on delayed X-rays, then open reduction internal fixation with or without bone graft is needed.

Boxer's (fifth metacarpal) fracture

This is a fracture of the neck of the fifth metacarpal secondary to direct trauma of a fist (punching a hard surface). This injury can be complicated with an open wound, which needs to be addressed in a timely manner to avoid infection.

Treatment –– This fracture is usually only treated with an ulnar splint and early mobilization, but significant displacement and angulation in this injury might warrant closed reduction or percutaneous K-wires, or even open reduction internal fixation (ORIF) of the metacarpal. Antibiotics should be prescribed if there is an associated wound over the knuckle as this should be assumed to be a fight bite until proven otherwise. This might need formal washout.

Neck-of-femur fracture

These are common in the elderly secondary to a fall. There is a high risk in patients with osteoporosis. Patients are unable to bear weight after the fall and present with a shortened and externally rotated leg. These injuries are divided into intracapsular and extracapsular fractures. Patients should have prophylaxis for deep vein thrombosis (this includes any lower limb injuries that leads to any period of immobilization) and consider bisphosphonate.

Treatment –– Generally, an intracapsular fracture if displaced requires a hemiarthroplasty or a total hip replacement if the patient is an appropriate candidate, as there is a high risk of avascular necrosis secondary to the disruption of the femoral head blood supply (predominantly the trochanteric anastomosis). If the fracture is undisplaced and the patient would be able to be compliant then fixation should be considered. A dynamic hip screw (DHS) or intramedullary device is the treatment of choice for extracapsular neck of femur fractures (see pp. 118–122).

Soft tissue knee injuries

These may be multiple injuries and commonly occur during sporting activities in non-contact twisting or hyperextension injuries.

Anterior cruciate ligament (ACL) -- This is a non-contact twisting injury to the knee with a degree of forced hyperextension or direct impact on an extended knee. Immediate swelling of the knee is common, owing to the vascularized ACL and a rupture causes an immediate haemarthrosis. Isolated ACL injury is not painful at the time. Commonly this injury is present with a meniscal and medial collateral ligament injury. The patient would present with acute swelling but progress to symptoms of instability. Examination of a ruptured ACL would show an acutely swollen knee, with positive Lachman's and anterior drawer test results, as well as a pivot shift test if the patient is compliant and able to relax for the examination. Treatment of ACL ruptures is either conservative with physiotherapy and rehabilitation, or ACL reconstruction using an autograft (hamstring or patella tendon), allograft or synthetic grafts.

Posterior cruciate ligament (PCL) -- This is a forced hyperextension injury. Examination reveals a positive posterior drawer test result. Treatment is usually conservative if the injury is in isolation but might require reconstruction if part of a multiligament injury.

Meniscal injury -- This results from acute twisting injury to the knee and also frequently presents as degenerative tears in elderly and arthritic knees. Swelling classically occurs hours after the acute injury. Clicking, locking and giving way are some of the symptoms of a meniscal tear. Pain on going up and down stairs is common, as is pain during hyperflexion. Examination findings include joint line tenderness and positive McMurray's test results on the side of the tear. Treatment can be conservative or operative with debridement or repair (if it is an acute tear in the peripheral third of the meniscus, which is vascularized).

Collateral ligaments -- Medial and lateral collateral ligament injuries usually occur in addition to one of the previous injuries. They are commonly a sprain injury as opposed to a complete rupture (this would indicate high-energy trauma). Examination would show opening of the joint in varus or valgus stress tests. Treatment is usually conservative with splinting, and the ligaments usually scar up.

Tibial fracture

This results from a direct trauma to the leg, usually with a degree of energy, either during sporting activities or in a road-traffic accident. The patient needs to be monitored for compartment syndrome if the fracture is a closed injury. The fracture may be open and should be dealt with in the standard manner.

Treatment -- Treatment is non-operative in a cast, if the fracture is minimally displaced. Operative management includes open reduction internal fixation (ORIF) with a plate and interfragmentary screws, intramedullary nail or an external fixator, especially in multifragmentory tibial fractures involving the tibial plafond or open fractures.

Achilles' tendon rupture

A complete or partial tear of the Achilles' tendon (gastrocnemius tendon complex) may occur anywhere from the musculo-tendonous junction to its attachment at the calcaneum. Ruptures occur from high stresses or force through the tendon, commonly in sporting activities that involve a forceful push-off with the foot. The patient usually presents with sudden severe pain in the back of the ankle that felt like a sharp physical blow and often might describe hearing a 'pop'. Examination with a Simmonds' test reveals absent plantar flexion. Palpation of the tendon often reveals a gap within a tendon and pain at the site of rupture.

Treatment -- This involves either non-operative treatment using sequential casting from plantar flexion to neutral position over six to nine weeks. Alternatively, surgical repair can be selected, with an increased risk of infection due to the lack of vascularity in that region but decreased chances of re-rupture (~3% vs. ~13%).

Ankle fracture

Most traumatic injuries to the ankle result in ankle sprain. Ankle fractures are usually caused by a direct fall or a twisting injury to the joint. Symptoms including immediate swelling, pain, deformity and inability to bear weight. It is important to identify whether the fracture is a lateral, medial or posterior malleolar fracture – this would be delineated on X-rays – and to determine whether there is any talar shift within the joint, as this would dictate the method of treatment.

Treatment -- Treatment is non-operative with a well-moulded cast if the fracture is undisplaced. If there is evidence of an unstable configuration or evidence of talar shift, treatment would usually involve open reduction internal fixation (ORIF).

Hip examination

The principles in the general examination section should be a guideline for each orthopaedic examination.

Clinical condition likely to be examined: osteoarthritis

The hip should be examined while the patient standing, walking and lying down.

Inspection

Expose the patient's lower limbs, leaving the underwear on. Start your examination with the patient standing, and inspect the hips from the front, side and back.

Skin
- Colour – any discolouration of the skin or bruising,
- Scars – surgical (lateral, posterior) vs. non-surgical,
- Sinuses – any visible discharge.

Shape
- Swelling – localized or diffuse,
- Asymmetry of skin creases,
- Muscle wasting.

Posture
- Increase in lumbar lordosis, scoliosis,
- Pelvic tilt,
- Limb shortening (to be measured when patient lying down),
- Fixed flexion deformity.

Trendelenburg's test –– This is to assess the hip abductors – stand facing the patient and support the patient with having his or her palms lying on your own. Ask the patient to stand on the good leg and flex the other leg off the floor and repeat with the bad leg. Note any sagging of the pelvis. The test is positive on the opposite side that sags, indicating weakness of the abductors (Figure 7.1).

While the patient is standing, you could continue to examine the patient's gait or leave it until the end. Then carry out inspection and the rest of the examination while the patient is lying down.

Gait
- Ask the patient to walk to the end of the room and back, observing the initiation of gait, the swing and the stance phases of the gait cycle.
- Observe the patient to detect any evidence of pain while walking in an antalgic gait.
- Observe the pelvis for a Trendelenburg's gait, e.g. where the pelvis of the left side dips when the left leg is lifted off the floor, indicating weakness in the hip abductors of the right side.

Inspection lying down
- Inspect for fixed flexion deformity.
- Inspect for obvious shortening and measure the real and apparent leg length using a tape measure, starting with the good leg and comparing the bad leg against it.
- Measure the apparent leg length: place the legs in a parallel position and run a tape measure from a fixed midline point such as the umbilicus to the medial

Table 7.1 Gait analysis

Gait	Cause	Clinically
Antalgic	Pain	Shortened stance phase and increased swing phase
Trendelenburg's	Deficient abductors	When the foot comes off the floor, the ipsilateral hip dips down instead of lifting up, owing to abductor deficiency on the other side
Parkinsonian	Parkinson's disease	Shuffling, small steps Forward flexed posture
Ataxic	Cerebellar lesion	Broad-based posture with a lurching quality, difficulty walking in straight line and turning
Short leg	Congenital (shortening of the femur or tibia) or acquired (e.g., fracture or proximally migrated hip osteoarthritis)	Ipsilateral hip drops when bearing weight on the short leg
High stepping	Foot drop (sciatic or common peroneal nerve palsy)	Foot slaps onto the ground, striking the sole of the foot instead of the heel
Spastic or scissor	Neurological cause, e. g., MS or cerebral palsy	Foot usually in equinus, with scissoring hips (in adduction)

malleolus. Fixed abduction will give you increased apparent length on the affected side, while fixed adduction will give a decreased apparent leg length.

- Measure the real leg length: place the pelvis 'square' onto the couch, i.e. at 90° to the body's long axis. Place the tape measure on the anterior superior iliac spine (ASIS), and measure to the medial malleolus. Any discrepancy in comparing both sides would indicate a real leg length discrepancy. You need to determine whether this is coming from the hip, femur or tibia.

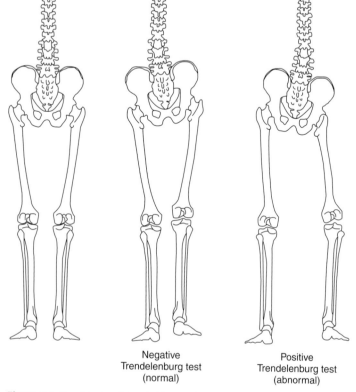

Negative
Trendelenburg test
(normal)

Positive
Trendelenburg test
(abnormal)

Figure 7.1 Trendelenburg's test in hip examination.

Palpation

Skin
- Temperature,
- Texture of skin.

Given that the hip joint is deep within the tissue, palpation is limited. You could palpate the greater trochanter for any tenderness, which might indicate trochanteric bursitis.

Movement

Before initiating the movements of the hip, it is wise to carry out Thomas' test for fixed flexion deformity.

Thomas' test

- Begin by placing one hand under the patient's lumbar spine, to detect the elimination of the lumbar lordosis by assisting the patient to flex both hips and knees.
- Ask the patient to extend the good hip fully, while maintaining the flexion of the contralateral hip with both patient's hands on the knee.
- Ensure that the lumbar lordosis flattening is maintained.
- Assess any residual fixed flexion of the extended leg and repeat with the affected hip.
- The fixed flexion is measured from the horizontal.

Flexion – 140° -- Active and passive hip flexion should be assessed using Thomas' test, by asking the patient to flex all the way up to the abdomen and stressing that hip to see whether any passive flexion can be achieved.

Internal rotation – 40° and external rotation – 40° -- With the hip flexed at 90°, one hand holding the foot and the other on the knee, assess the rotation by moving the foot laterally (internal rotation) and medially (external rotation). This should be repeated with the leg extended.

Abduction – 45° and adduction – 30° -- Grasp the heel of the leg with one hand and place the other hand on the anterior superior iliac spine (ASIS), move the leg laterally (abduction) and medially towards and crossing the midline (adduction). The hand on the ASIS detects any pelvic tilt, which would give a discrepancy in measurement.

Crepitus -- This should be listened for and palpated on all joint movements.

Neurovascular examination

- Power – MRC scale M0–M5: each muscle group,
- Sensation: neurology of limb,
- Distal pulses: anterior tibial, posterior tibial and dorsalis pedis pulses,
- Reflexes of lower limb.

For completion

- Examine the back and knee.
- Review X-rays of the pelvis and hip (anteroposterior and lateral).

Features of osteoarthritis: LOSS

- Loss of joint space,
- Osteophyte formation,
- Subchondral sclerosis,
- Subchondral cysts.

Tips and hints

- In hip osteoarthritis, early features include restricted movements in internal and external rotation, abduction and adduction.
- There are no specific blood markers for osteoarthritis; diagnosis is made through history, examination and radiographs.

Knee examination

The principles in the general examination section should be a guideline for each orthopaedic examination.

Most common case: knee osteoarthritis

It is probably best to start your examination by observing the patient walking.

- Comment on the gait (see hip examination) – antalgic gait, stiff-leg gait, varus thrust.
- Observe for genu valgum or varum.

Inspection

Look around the bed for special footwear and walking aids.

Skin

- Colour – any discolouration of the skin, bruising or erythema,
- Scars – surgical vs. non-surgical, arthroscopic portals,
- Sinuses – any visible discharge.

Shape

- Swelling – localized or diffuse (intra- or extra-articular); baker's cyst – swelling in the popliteal fossa,
- Quadriceps muscle wasting (the circumference can be measured and compared with the contralateral leg),
- Bony or soft tissue prominences or deformities.

Symmetry

- Alignment:
  - Genu varus or valgus (varus and fixed flexion is commonly seen in osteoarthritis),
  - Fixed flexion or hyperextension.
- Bilateral or unilateral deformities.

Palpation

Skin

- Temperature (using the dorsum of the hand),
- Texture of skin.

Soft tissue, effusion

- Soft tissue masses – shape, size, position, consistency, fluctuation.
- Patellar tap: this test is used for moderate effusions. While compressing the suprapatellar pouch with one hand, press the anterior aspect of the patella downwards. If the patella can be felt to bounce off the femoral condyles, effusions are present.
- Patella bulge test: this test is more sensitive for small effusions; however, if the patella tap test was positive this test is not required. Start by emptying the medial parapatellar retinacular area by pressing your hand and 'milking' the joint upwards towards the suprapatellar pouch. Then sweep your hand from superior to inferior along the lateral aspect of the knee. If an effusion is present, you will observe a fluid ripple or 'bulge' appear on the medial aspect of the knee.

Joints and bones –– Check for tenderness, either localized or diffuse; comparison is crucial.

- Palpate with one finger around the patella margins with the knee in extension.
- Grind test of the patella: move the patella superiorly and inferiorly while applying downward pressure against the trochlea and femur. Pain exhibited during this manoeuvre indicates patellofemoral osteoarthritis.
- Palpate the medial and lateral joint line with the knee in 90° of flexion: palpate over the patella tendon and tibial tubercle, medial collateral ligament (MCL) and lateral collateral ligament (LCL), as well as the popliteal fossa.
- At this 90°-flexed position, assess for 'posterior sag', by looking across both knees flexed together from the side. A 'sag' sign is present if the tibia of the affected side 'drops back', indicating a posterior cruciate ligament injury (PCL).

Movement

Both active and passive movements should be assessed. Pain and restriction in any movement should be noted and compared with the other side.

Ensure that you do not cause any pain to the patient during any part of the examination, and always explain to the patient what you are about to do or test (this especially applies with patients with painful arthritic knees).

- Begin by making a quick assessment of the quadriceps muscles by asking the patient to raise the leg, keeping it straight; at this point, you could also assess the power of the quads.
- Assess for extension and hyperextension by cupping the patient's heel and asking the patient to relax. Note whether any hyperextension occurs. If no hyperextension is present, then the range of movement starts from 0°.

- Ask the patient to flex the knee as far as possible with your hand on the patient's knee, feeling for any clicking or crepitus during movement. Once the patient reaches the maximum flexion, attempt to take it further passively, to aim for the calf to touch the hamstrings and thus achieving a flexion of 140°. Make a note of the passive and active degrees of flexion if a difference is present.

Special tests

Collateral ligaments

Varus and valgus stress tests	With the patient's foot tucked between your arm and chest, flex the knee to 20–30° and then apply a varus and valgus stress with your free hand on the knee to assess the amount of joint opening upon stressing it. Pain or opening of the medial joint line on valgus stress, or lateral joint on varus stress, indicates a sprain or tear to the medial or lateral collateral ligament, respectively.

Cruciate ligaments

Anterior drawer	The test is performed to assess the anterior cruciate ligament with the knee flexed to 90° in a supine patient. The examiner sits on the patient's foot and grasps the knee with both hands, thumbs placed over the tibial plateau. An anterior force is applied. The amount of tibial translation anteriorly is compared with that on the contralateral side (Figure 7.2).
Posterior drawer	This test is performed to assess the posterior cruciate ligament. This is the same test as the anterior drawer test but instead of an anterior force, a posterior force is applied to the tibia and the posterior translation in comparison with the contralateral side is noted.

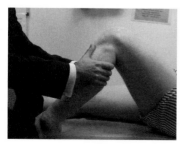

Figure 7.2 Anterior drawer test in knee examination.

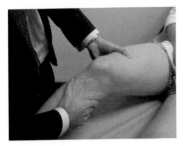

Figure 7.3 Lachman's test in knee examination.

a
b

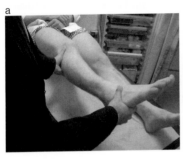

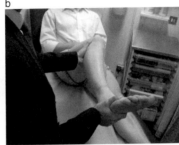

Figure 7.4 Pivot shift in knee examination: (a) fully extended knee; (b) translation of the tibia as knee begins to flex.

Lachman's test	The knee is placed in 20–30° of flexion. The femur is stabilized with the non-dominant hand. An anteriorly placed force is applied to the proximal tibia with the dominant hand. The amount of translation of the tibia on the femur, and the firmness of the 'endpoint' should be compared with that of the contralateral knee. This is the most sensitive test to detect an ACL injury (Figure 7.3).
Pivot shift	In the fully extended ACL-deficient knee, the tibia is reduced relative to the femur (Figure 7.4a). As the knee begins to flex, gravity results in translation of the tibia (Figure 7.4b). At ~40° of flexion, the translation reduces, resulting in 'shifting or pivoting' of the tibia into its correct alignment with the femur. This 'jumping' is due to the iliotibial band falling behind the axis of rotation of the femur. The pivot shift test is best performed with the patient fully relaxed. The leg is extended, the foot in internal rotation, and a valgus stress is applied to the tibia.

Menisci

McMurray's test	This test helps identify a meniscal tear in the medial or lateral compartments. This test can be uncomfortable or painful and examiners often stop you from proceeding once you mention that this would be the next test you would want to perform. To test the medial meniscus, you would flex the knee maximally and apply one hand on the posteromedial joint line and the other on the foot. Whilst in that position, externally rotate the foot and extend the knee, palpating for a click or pain to suggest a meniscal tear. To assess the lateral meniscus, palpate the posterolateral joint line and internally rotate the foot undergoing the same movements as for the medial side.

For completion

- Assess the neurovascular status of the limb.
- Review anteroposterior, lateral, skyline (patellofemoral joint) or Rosenberg views (assess the joint space more accurately) of the knee, and weight-bearing status.
- Examine the hip and ankle.

Foot examination

The principles in the general examination section should be a guideline for each orthopaedic examination.

Scenarios that should be considered in the examination include:

- Hallux valgus,
- Hallux rigidus,
- Hammer-toes,
- Claw toes,
- Pes cavus and planus,
- Charcot's foot.

Inspection

Look around the bed for shoes (inspect footwear inside and on the sole) and walking aids.

Skin

- Colour – Any discolouration of the skin or bruising or erythema,
- Scars – Surgical vs. non-surgical,
- Sinuses – Any visible discharge.

Nails
- Pitting,
- Spooning,
- Clubbing,
- Paronychia,

Shape
- Swelling – localized or diffuse,
- Muscle wasting,
- Bony or soft tissue prominences or deformities: hallux valgus, hammer-toes, claw toes, retracted second toe, over-riding fifth toe,
- Corns and callosities over the joints and on the plantar surface indicate pressure points,

Symmetry
- Bilateral or unilateral deformities.

It might be advisable to observe the patient walking at this point including some test:

- Observe both feet at the same time with patient standing and walking (e.g. foot drop due to nerve injury).
- Observe the patient walking on tiptoe (foot plantarflexion) and on the heels (dorsiflexion), assessing S1–2 and L4–5, respectively.
- Ask the patient to stand on tiptoes. Observe for varus position of the hindfoot – best seen from behind.
- With the patient standing one foot in front of the other, assess the ankle position and the integrity of the medial, lateral and transverse arches. Inspect for the 'too many toes' sign, also observed from behind, which indicates tibialis posterior dysfunction.

Palpation

Skin
- Temperature,
- Texture of skin.

Joints and bones
- Tenderness – localized or diffuse; comparison is crucial,
- Bony prominences – lateral and medial malleoli,
- Foot bones – os calcis, tarsal bones and metatarsals (including joints).

Soft tissue, ligaments and tendons
- Soft tissue masses – shape, size, position, consistency, fluctuation,
- Achilles' tendon (palpate along the tendon for any tenderness or defect),

- Palpation along the peroneal tendons posterior to the lateral malleolus,
- Palpation along the tibialis posterior tendon posterior to the medial malleolus,
- Palpation of the plantar surface including the fascia, heel, fifth metatarsal, evidence of a Morton's neuroma in the plantar web spaces.
- Squeeze test of the metatarsals for tenderness and subluxation of the metatarsophalangeal joint (in rheumatoid arthritis).

Movement

Both active and passive movements should be assessed. Pain and restriction in any movement should be noted and compared with the other side.

- Plantar flexion and dorsiflexion of the ankle joint,
- Inversion and eversion of the subtalar joint,
- Supination and pronation, abduction and adduction of the midtarsal joint,
- Flexion and extension of the metatarsophalangeal joint and interphalangeal joints,
- Inversion and eversion of the foot passively and actively against resistance (palpating for the tibialis posterior tendon and peroneal tendons, respectively).

Neurovascular examination

Motor
- Assess muscles on the MRC (0–5) scale.

Sensation
- Sural nerve: laterally,
- Deep and superficial peroneal nerves,
- Medial and lateral plantar nerves.

Distal pulses
- Anterior tibial pulse: midway between the medial and lateral malleoli,
- Posterior tibial pulse: posterior to medial malleolus,
- Dorsal pedis pulse: on dorsum of foot in the first web space, lateral to the extensor hallucis longus,
- Check for capillary refill <2 seconds.

Special tests

Not all of these tests are expected to be completed. They should be tailored to your initial clinical findings and suspicions.

Simmonds' test	Squeeze test of the gastrocnemius producing plantar flexion – if absent then an Achilles' tendon rupture is suspected.

Anterior drawer test	To assess the ankle joint stability.
Tinel's test	To investigate tarsal tunnel syndrome by percussing the posterior tibial nerve (posterior to the medial malleolus). Sharp pain and numbness caused by percussion supports the diagnosis.
Test for tibialis posterior dysfunction	The patient would be unable to stand on a single foot tiptoe on the affected leg, or contract the tibialis posterior in the plantar-flexed inverted position against resistance.

Common toe deformities to note

Hallux valgus	Visible valgus deformity with bunion present. On X-ray: assess degree of valgus deformity; first or second intermetatarsal angle; distal metatarsal articular angle; presence of osteoarthritis in the first metatarsophalangeal joint.
Hammer toes	Most common on the second toe; may be associated with hallux valgus. The distal interphalangeal joint can be in any position but is most commonly in extension.
Claw toes	Commonly affects all lesser toes and may be bilateral; flexion deformity at proximal and distal interphalangeal joints (in contrast to hammer toes); callosities common; check if fixed or mobile deformities. Can be associated with neurological pathology.

For completion

- Always ask to examine the patient's shoes, as these give the clinician ample information about the deformities, alignment and weight-bearing points during walking.
- Review X-rays of the ankle (anteroposterior and lateral) and foot (weight-bearing anteroposterior, oblique and lateral).
- Examine the knee, hip and spine.

Shoulder examination

The principles in the general examination section should be a guideline for each orthopaedic examination.

Probable clinical conditions to be examined: rotator cuff tear, shoulder osteoarthritis, impingement syndrome and frozen shoulder (the latter two are painful conditions and therefore less likely).

Inspection

Have the patient sitting in the middle of the room with both shoulders visible, so anterior and posterior inspection is possible.

Skin
- Colour – Any discolouration of the skin or bruising,
- Scars – Surgical vs. non-surgical,
- Sinuses – Any visible discharge.

Shape
- Swelling – localized or diffuse,
- Bony or soft tissue prominences,
- Posture,

Symmetry

Muscle wasting	Loss of shoulder contour due to proximal myopathy of the deltoid; above the spine of the scapula from supraspinatus wasting, and below the spine of the scapula from infraspinatus wasting.
Testing serratus anterior	Ask patient to push hands against the wall: look for winging of the scapula; this indicates a long thoracic nerve palsy.

Palpation

Skin
- Temperature,
- Texture of skin.

Joint
- Tenderness – localized or diffuse; comparison is crucial as some sites are tender in normal circumstances.
- Ask patient to lift arm – feel the shaft and humeral head via the axilla.
- Bony prominences – palpate medial to lateral. Check: sternoclavicular joint (SCJ), clavicle (deformity due to previous fracture), acromioclavicular joint (ACJ) (any subluxation or dissociation), acromion and coracoid.
- Feel the anterior and lateral aspects of glenohumeral joint and the greater tuberosity.
- Swelling – localized or diffuse: within the joint (synovial effusion, haemarthrosis, pyarthrosis) or extending beyond the joint (infections, tumours, lymphatic or venous drainage disruptions).
- Soft tissue masses – shape, size, position, consistency, fluctuation.

Movement

Before examining the shoulder, it would be prudent to conduct a screening examination of the neck, asking the patient to touch chin to chest, extend the neck, turn towards the left and right, and report whether there is any pain.

Stand opposite the patient and assess active movements by asking the patient to imitate your movements. Always compare against the good side and test passive movements.

Abduction – 170° 'Lift both your arms out to the side slowly. Can your shoulders touch your ears?'

- Initiation of abduction (predominantly glenohumeral). Difficulty or pain indicates a rotator cuff tear.
- Painful arc 60°–120°: consider impingement syndrome (rotator cuff or supraspinatus tendonitis) or partial cuff tear.
- Painful arc 140°–170°: consider acromioclavicular joint osteoarthritis.

Adduction – ~50°	'Move your arm straight across your chest.'
Forward Flexion – ~165°	'Lift both arms forward together as far as you can take them.'
Extension – ~60°	
External rotation at 90° elbow flexion – 90°	'Press your elbows onto your chest and copy my movement.' Difficulty in external rotation can indicate a frozen shoulder or infraspinatus or teres minor pathology.
Internal rotation at 90° elbow flexion – T6–T8	'Put your hand behind your back. How far up can you reach with your thumb?'
Crepitus	Across the glenohumeral joint and the acromioclavicular joint.

Neurovascular examination

Moter	MRC scale M0–M5: deltoid power in abduction against resistance,
Sensory	Axillary nerve palsy results in decreased sensation in the 'regimental badge' region,
Distal pulses	Brachial and radial pulses.

Special tests

Not all these tests are expected to be completed. They should be tailored to your initial clinical findings and suspicions.

Rotator cuff muscles can be tested individually to delineate where the pathology is arising from – pain indicates tendonitis, while weakness is associated with a tear. The muscles of the rotator cuff can be remembered using SITS: supraspinatus, infraspinatus, teres minor, subscapularis.

Supraspinatus	With the elbow in extension, and the arm in full internal rotation, 20° of abduction and forward flexion – test for resisted abduction. A tear in the supraspinatus would prevent initiation of abduction.
Infraspinatus or teres minor	With the elbow in 90° of flexion – test for resisted external rotation.
Subscapularis	Gerber's 'lift-off' test – elbow in 90° flexion and internally rotated behind the back, with an attempt at resisted lift-off from the back.
Biceps	A tear in the long head of biceps can be delineated pain or weakness on resisted flexion of the elbow and with supination (distal tear), showing a 'Popeye' bulge.

For completion

- Examine the neck and elbow.
- Review X-rays of the shoulder.

Tips and hints

- Intra-articular disease causes pain in most shoulder movements, whereas tendonitis usually causes pain in one specific direction (e.g. supraspinatus tendonitis in abduction).
- Neurological lesions and complete tendon ruptures cause painless and weak or no movements in the specific direction of action.

Hand and wrist examination

The principles in the general examination section should be a guideline for each orthopaedic examination.

Scenarios that should be considered in the examination include:

- Dupuytren's contracture,
- Carpal tunnel syndrome,
- Rheumatoid arthritis in the hands,
- Osteoarthritis in the hands,
- Mallet finger,
- Trigger finger,
- Brachial plexus injury,

- Ulnar nerve lesion,
- Radial nerve lesion.

Inspection

Observe both hands at the same time with the patient sitting down and the hands placed on a pillow or table.

Skin
- Colour – any discolouration of the skin or bruising,
- Scars – surgical vs. non-surgical,
- Sinuses – any visible discharge.

Nails
- Pitting,
- Spooning,
- Clubbing,
- Paronychia.

Shape
- Swelling, localized or diffuse,
- Bony or soft tissue prominences,
- Nodules,
- Deformities: swan neck deformity, boutonniere deformity, mallet finger.

Symmetry
- Asymmetry – e.g., ulnar deviation of fingers,
- Muscle wasting – loss of thenar or hypothenar eminence, interosseous muscle wasting.

Palpation

Skin
- Temperature,
- Texture of skin.

Joints and bones

Tenderness	Localized or diffuse; comparison is crucial as some sites are tender in normal circumstances.
Bony prominences	Radial styloid, ulnar styloid, metacarpophalangeal joint, proximal and distal interphalangeal joints.
Swelling	Localized or diffuse: within joint (synovial effusion, haemarthrosis, pyarthrosis) or extending

beyond the joint (infections, tumours, lymphatic or venous drainage disruptions).

Anatomical snuffbox	Located distal and dorsal to the radial styloid, bordered by abductor pollicis longus (APL) and extensor pollicis brevis (EPB) on radial side, and extensor pollicis longus (EPL) on the ulnar side. The cephalic vein and the deep branch of the radial artery can often be palpated. The scaphoid represents the floor of the anatomical snuffbox. Tenderness on palpation suggests fracture of the scaphoid (see p. 89).
Distal interphalangeal joints (DIPJ)	Heberden's nodes indicate osteoarthritis.
Proximal interphalangeal joints (PIPJ)	Bouchard's nodes indicate osteoarthritis.

Soft tissue

Abductor pollicis longus (APL) and extensor pollicis brevis (EPB)	Tenderness at the site of the tendon may indicate stenosing tenosynovitis (De Quervain's disease).
Ganglion	A round, pea-sized, cystic, jelly-like swelling, found on the dorsal or volar aspect of the wrist. Mobile and non-tender on palpation with no deep soft tissue or muscular attachments.
Thenar and hypothenar eminence	Wasting is seen at the base of the thumb or little finger, respectively. The former occurs in median nerve compression (CTS) and the latter in compression of the ulnar nerve.
Palmaris longus (PL)	The presence of this tendon should be determined (it is absent in 15% of population); it is an important landmark as well as a source of tendon graft. Wrist flexion with opposition of the thumb to the little finger allows the midline tendon to become prominent. It is ulnar to flexor carpi radialis (FCR).
Palpation of the palm	Look for any nodules along the tendons or thickening (Dupuytren's disease).

| Soft tissue masses | Shape, size, position, consistency, fluctuation. |

Movement

Both active and passive movements should be assessed indicating degrees or arc of movement. Pain and restriction in any movement should be noted and compared with the other side.

| Flexor digitorum superficialis | Tested by active flexion of the finger while holding other fingers in hyperextension. |
| Flexor digitorum profundus | Tested by fixing the intermediate phalanx and flexing the distal interphalangeal joint in isolation. |

Thumb

- Check opposition to all fingers in turn.
- Test the extensor pollicis longus by asking the patient to lift the thumb up off a table whilst the hand is held palm down on the table.

Neurovascular examination

Motor
- Power MRC scale, M0–M5.
- Myotomes:
  - Wrist extension: C6,
  - Wrist flexion: C7,
  - Finger extension: C7,
  - Finger flexion: C8,
  - Finger abduction and adduction: T1.
- Nerve distribution:
  - Median nerve: test thumb abduction; 'OK' sign of thumb to index opposition tests anterior interosseus nerve (AIN).
  - Ulnar nerve: test finger abduction, using Froment's test. The patient grasps a piece of paper between the thumb and index finger. The examiner attempts to pull the paper away. If the patient is forced to flex the tip of the thumb to maintain grip, the test is positive, i.e. ulnar nerve palsy is present.
  - Radial nerve and posterior interosseus nerve: test wrist and finger extension.

Sensation
- Dermatomes:
  - Thumb and index finger: C6,
  - Middle finger: C7,
  - Ring and little finger: C8.

- Autonomous nerve areas:
  - Radial nerve: dorsal aspect of first web space,
  - Median nerve: volar aspect of the tip of the index finger,
  - Ulnar nerve: volar aspect of the tip of the little finger.

Distal pulses –– radial and ulnar artery and capillary refill.

Special tests

Not all these tests are expected to be completed. They should be tailored to your initial clinical findings and suspicions.

Phalen's test	Place the dorsum of both hands in full palmar flexion. This should be held for a minute. If median nerve compression (carpal tunnel syndrome) is present, symptoms of numbness in the median nerve distribution will occur.
Tinel's test	Tap onto the palmar area overlying the median nerve (mid proximal palmar crease), which may produce a tingling sensation along the median nerve distribution in carpal tunnel syndrome.
Finkelstein's test	Have the patient make a fist with the thumb tucked in full flexion, and the fist in ulnar deviation. Pain radially indicates De Quervain's tenosynovitis.
Froment's test	As before.

For completion

- Examine the shoulder and elbow.
- Review X-rays of the wrist (anteroposterior and lateral) and hand (anteroposterior, oblique and lateral).

Spinal examination – lumbar spine

The principles in the general examination section should be a guideline for each orthopaedic examination.

The most common case would be lumbar disc herniation or spinal stenosis. Expect to find some focal neurological deficit in your examination: it is paramount that you are gentle in the examination to avoid causing the patient any pain.

With the patient exposed but in underwear, start the examination with the patient facing you.

Gait

Observe the patient's gait, noting evidence of an antalgic gait, or any other gait pattern that might indicate pain or concurrent lower limb pathology. Patients with back pain often walk leaning forwards in a partially flexed posture to off-load the pressure on the lumbar spine.

Inspection

Look around the bed for walking aids. Inspect the patient while standing: from front, side and back.

Skin
- Colour – Any discolouration of the skin, bruising, erythema or café au lait spots or nodules (neurofibromas),
- Scars – Surgical vs. non-surgical.

Shape and symmetry
- General posture.
- Pelvic tilt, leg length discrepancy.
- Muscle symmetry; comparing left to right, and proximal to distal.
- Atrophy and wasting of muscle (upper and lower limbs).
- Alignment of spine; straight or evidence of scoliosis (lateral curvature with rotational deformity of vertebral bodies).
- Note the cervical, thoracic and lumbar curves – commenting on any loss or exaggeration of kyphosis or lordosis. This is best assessed from the side.
- To detect any subtle fixed flexion you could try the *wall test* by asking the patient to stand with the back against a wall. Ensure that heels, buttocks, shoulders and head touch the wall.

Palpation

- Palpate the spine from cervical to lumbar.
- Palpate the spinous processes noting any bony tenderness, or any prominence or step.
- Palpate the left and right paravertebral muscles.

Movement

Ensure that you do not cause any pain to the patient during any point of the examination, and always communicate with the patient what you are about to do or examine.

Flexion –– Ensure that you are assessing spinal rather than hip flexion by marking two points ~10 cm apart on the midline of the lumbar spine. Ask the patient to touch the toes: the points should separate by a further ~5 cm on flexion.

- If scoliosis is present, flexion will accentuate curvature by causing a rib prominence, like a hump, on the convexity of the spinal curve and a skin crease on its concavity.

- However, if the apparent scoliosis disappears on forward flexion, it is postural.
- If the scoliosis disappears on sitting, it may be due to limb length discrepancy.

Extension –– Normally this is 30°. Ask the patient to arch backwards, but note that patients who get pain on doing this might bend their knees to compensate.

Lateral flexion –– Ask the patient to slide a hand down the ipsilateral thigh on one side, and then down the other. Although you would expect 30° of lateral flexion, asymmetry is more relevant clinically.

Rotation –– Most rotation occurs at the thoracic spine. Lumbo sacral pathology should not affect rotation. This is best assessed with the patient sitting down (to fix the pelvis) and having the patient fold the hands and rotate to each side. Note any asymmetry of range of movement. This has limited clinical relevance.

Supine

- Observe the patient getting on the couch.
- Neurological examination of the lower limbs:
  - Tone.
  - Sensation. Assess each dermatome with light touch (see Figure 5.6). Further sensory examination should include pin prick, two-point discrimination vibration and temperature.
  - Power. Test each movement in the lower limb: hip flexion and extension, knee flexion and extension, ankle dorsiflexion and plantar flexion and extension of the big toe (extensor hallucis longus). This should be a measure on the MRC power scale (0–5).
  - Reflexes: knee, ankle and plantar reflexes (Babinski's reflex).
  - Findings of these neurological tests should be collected, to establish which nerve root is involved in the lumbar spine pathology.
- Straight leg raise (SLR): with the knee extended, have the patient passively flex the hip by lifting the heel off the couch and estimate the angle at which pain or discomfort occurs (normally 80°). Pain radiating from back towards the knee, calf and down to ankle and foot is suggestive of sciatic nerve root irritation. Hamstring tightness is not clinically significant. Note: if the SLR of the unaffected contralateral leg causes pain in the symptomatic leg (cross SLR) then this is a specific sign of lumbar disc herniation.

- Sciatic stretch test: with the patient's hip and knee fully extended, tension on the sciatic nerve can be increased by ankle dorsiflexion, causing an increase in pain. This is relieved by flexing the knee.

Waddell's non-organic signs

Always think of Waddell's non-organic signs (psychological component to lower back pain):[1]

Superficial or non-anatomical tenderness	Lightly pinch the skin on a wide area of lumbar skin (pinch test). If this causes pain, test is positive.
Axial loading	Vertical loading with the palm of the hand against the patient's head. If this causes pain, the test is positive.
Distraction	If severe pain is exhibited on a straight leg raise, but the patient is able to sit comfortably forward and upright with legs extended on the examination couch, this test is positive.
Regional disturbances	The test is positive in presence of non-anatomical motor or sensory deficits (e.g. normal heel–toe walk, but cog-wheel foot weakness).
Over-reaction	The test is positive if muscle spasm, tremor or collapse occur during examination.

For completion

- Examine the patient prone, where you can carry out the femoral stretch test (straight leg raise, but extending straight leg as opposed to flexing).
- Assess the peripheral distal pulses.
- Perform a rectal examination, assessing anal tone and perianal sensation.
- Review anteroposterior and lateral X-rays of the spine (specifically the area in question, cervical, thoracic or lumbar. If cervical – ensure that you have views of the odontoid peg and that the lateral view reveals up to the T1 vertebra).
- Examine the shoulders, hip and knees, as relevant.

---

[1] G. Waddell, J. A. McCulloch, E. Kummel and R. M. Venner (1980) Nonorganic physical signs in low-back pain. *Spine* **5**:117–25.

Chapter # Clinical examinations (vascular)

Peripheral vascular examination

The patient will lie supine on the examination couch with the leg exposed from the hip to the foot.

The examination will follow the principle of *inspection, palpation and auscultation*. Further, specialized tests include Buerger's test, and measurement of the ankle–brachial pressure index (ABPI).

Inspection

Expose the patient's lower limbs, keeping underwear on. Start your examination with the patient standing, and inspect the legs from the front, side and back.

- Shiny hairless skin,
- Cellulitis,
- Arterial ulcers, especially on the toes,
- Venous ulcers, especially on the medial aspect of the tibia and medial malleolus,
- Peripheral oedema,
- Surgical scars, e.g. previous peripheral vascular surgery,
- Toes for dry gangrene,
- Do not forget to inspect the heels for ulcers.

Palpation

- Feel areas of erythema to distinguish simple dermatitis from infected cellulitis.
- Check the capillary refill of the toes: should be <3 seconds.
- Palpate pulses:
  - Femoral artery in the mid-inguinal point.
  - Popliteal artery, by flexing the knee and palpating the popliteal fossa. An aneurysm may also be felt.

- Posterior tibial behind the medial malleolus.
- Dorsalis pedis: lateral to the tendon of the extensor hallucis longus muscle.

Auscultation

For bruits over the femoral arteries.

Special tests

Buerger's test –– The patient's leg is elevated 45° and the colour of the foot is noted for over a minute. If the leg is chronically ischaemic, pallor will develop with a reactive hyperaemia once the leg is put down.

Ankle–brachial pressure index
- Systolic pressure in the ankle divided by systolic pressure in the arm, measured using a Doppler probe. A ratio of <0.5 indicates severe ischaemia.
- In the presence of calcification of the vessel wall, the reading maybe falsely high. This also applies to patients with diabetes.

Lower limb venous examination

Describe the surface anatomy of the long saphenous vein

The vein starts over the medial malleolus from the veins over the dorsum of the foot. It continues superiorly, over the medial aspect of the calf to the medial side of the knee joint, one hand's breadth posterior to the medial side of the joint. It continues superiorly along the medial side of the thigh and pierces the cribriform fascia at the saphenofemoral junction (SFJ).

What are the venous perforators? Where are they located?

These are venous channels connecting the superficial veins to the deep venous system. They play a role in recurrence of varicose veins if they are not controlled at the time of operation.

Locations are:
- *Hunterian* perforator: located in the mid-thigh,
- *Dodd* perforators in the distal thigh,
- *Boyd* perforators: around the knee down to mid calf,
- *Cockett's* perforators: located more posteriorly in the calf.

Patient examination

The patient examination is carried out with the patient initially standing and then supine, exposed from the hip to the foot.

The examination will follow the principle of inspection, palpation, auscultation and special tests.

Inspection (standing)

- Look at the distribution of the varicose veins, including posteriorly at the short saphenous system.
- Look at the saphenofemoral junction for the lump of a *saphena varix*.
- Look at the saphenofemoral junction for any scar from previous varicose vein surgery. Healed stab incisions may also be seen further down the leg.

Palpation (standing)

- Palpate the saphenofemoral junction for a *saphena varix*.
- Feel the distribution of varicose veins, which might not be immediately obvious on inspection.

Auscultation (standing)

Auscultate the saphenofemoral junction for a venous hum.

Inspection (supine)

- The varicose veins and any *saphena varix* will disappear.
- Look at the lower leg for venous eczema and venous ulcers, especially on the medial side over the tibia and anterior to the medial malleolus.

Palpation (supine)

- Palpation of the saphenofemoral junction confirms that the mass seen and felt is a *saphena varix* and not a *femoral hernia*.
- Palpate the skin around any ulcers to note if they might be infected with regional cellulitis.

Special test: tourniquet (Trendelenburg's) test

- The leg is elevated to drain the blood from the superficial venous system.
- A tourniquet is applied to the mid-thigh *below* the saphenofemoral junction (SFJ).
- The patient is asked to stand up.
- If the varicose veins re-appear below the tourniquet, it suggests that there are incompetent perforators below the SFJ.
- Incompetence at the SFJ causes the varicose veins to refill once the tourniquet is released.

Appendix: Additional high-yield topics for the MRCS

Further to the use of the chapters in this book as an aid for question-and-answer scenarios and practice with colleagues, here are a few more scenarios that may not be covered fully in independent chapters, which might be useful for consideration prior to the examination.

Surgical skills and patient safety

- Hand washing,
- Scrubbing for theatre and de-gowning,
- Insertion of urinary catheter,
- Intravenous cannulation, central venous pressure line (CVP) insertion, chest tube insertion, cricothyroidotomy: all with advanced trauma life support principles or scenarios,
- Suturing of laceration or excision biopsy of skin lesion (benign or malignant), including knowledge of margins and filling pathology forms,
- Postoperative analgesic ladder,
- Non-accidental injury in children – be aware of the signs.

Communication

- History of joint osteoarthritis – know the classic symptoms.
- History of lower back pain, radiating leg pain – differentiate between lumbar disc prolapse and spinal stenosis.
- History of limb claudication and ischaemia, and relevant investigations.
- Obtain patient consent for a hip or knee replacement as well as for treatment of a neck of femur fracture. Look out for the confused patient who may not be able to retain information or consent to an operation. Emergency procedures are different from elective cases. Consider the need for a mini mental state examination and discussion with family. Appreciate the different types of consent forms and the authority needed to obtain consent on behalf of a patient who lacks capacity.
- Order a theatre list with a selection of patients, including (some of): a child, MRSA-positive patient, elderly patient with a fractured neck of femur, diabetic patient, cardiac patient, patient with dirty wound or abscess. Discuss your reasoning.
- Refer an acutely ill patient to the intensive care unit or medical team. Refer a patient to the coroner. Inform your consultant of a multi-trauma patient

(consider open fracture management, blood loss, external fixation, vascular or plastic surgery input, transfer to specialist unit). Be aware of the key information that must be discussed, depending on the scenario.

- Counsel a patient regarding blood transfusion or regarding a needlestick injury, explaining the relevant blood test needed.
- Discuss a 'do not attempt resuscitation' (DNAR) status with patient and family.
- Break bad news: amputation; death; rheumatoid arthritis; paralysis secondary to cauda equina syndrome or cord compression.

Anatomy

- Review prosections of forearm, thigh, leg and foot, as well as the shoulder, hip, knee joints, popliteal fossa and antecubital fossa. Identify the main muscles with their insertions and their actions, and vessels and nerves and their innervations.
- Review bones: clavicle, humerus, carpal bones, hemi-pelvis, femur, patella, tibia, foot. Identify the side and orientation of the bone (left or right), grooves, tubercles, muscle attachments, arches (foot).

- Review the brachial plexus and injuries associated with it.
- Surface anatomy: anatomical snuffbox, upper limb and lower limb dermatomes.

Critical care

- Mechanism of action of anti-platelet medications and anti-coagulants, and how they affect the surgical patient pre- and postoperatively,
- Types of anaesthesia (methods, uses, complications),
- Pulmonary embolism or fat embolism post long bone fracture or postoperatively,
- Different types of fluid infusion and fluid management,
- Assessment and management of a burns patient: remember that fluid management is different in children.

Operative surgery

- Varicose veins and their management – conservative and operative,
- Ankle fracture open reduction internal fixation (Weber B),
- Distal radius fracture management: extra-articular, intra-articular; non-operative, MUA, K-wire, open reduction internal fixation.

Index